I0425637

COUCHESTHENTICS®
THE EXERCISE BOOK FOR PEOPLE WHO NEVER EXERCISE
BY
ROBERT SHAW

A simple manual of basic stretching and light-strength
exercises for men, women, and children

Copyright © 2012 by Robert Shaw

All rights reserved. No part of this book may be reproduced, stored, or transmitted
by any means—whether auditory, graphic, mechanical, or electronic—without
written permission of the author, except in the case of brief excerpts used in
critical articles and reviews. Unauthorized reproduction of any part
of this work is illegal and is punishable by law.

ISBN 978-1-105-98267-5

Printed in the United States of America

Cover Design and Photography by Robert Shaw
Marathon photo provided by ShutterStock

CouchEsthentics — Exercise: basic stretching and light strength
Health — For Men, Women and Children

CouchEsthentics® is a registered trademark of Hot & Glassy Productions

DISCLAIMER: I am not a doctor or a licensed physical trainer. I am a man who overcame
weight and fitness problems using these and other exercises in the comfort of my home.
There are warnings throughout this book concerning consulting your physician and
overexerting yourself. I take no responsibility for any injuries or ailments that might occur.

DEDICATION

This book is dedicated to my wonderful wife, Nancy, who has been the light of my life for more than twenty years. A woman of many talents and incredible intelligence, she has spent most of her working life behind a desk and has spent very little time exercising. I designed this simple regimen of low-key stretching and strength exercises for her and others to be able to remain in the comfort, privacy, and safety of their own homes and still get the exercise they need.

Robert Shaw

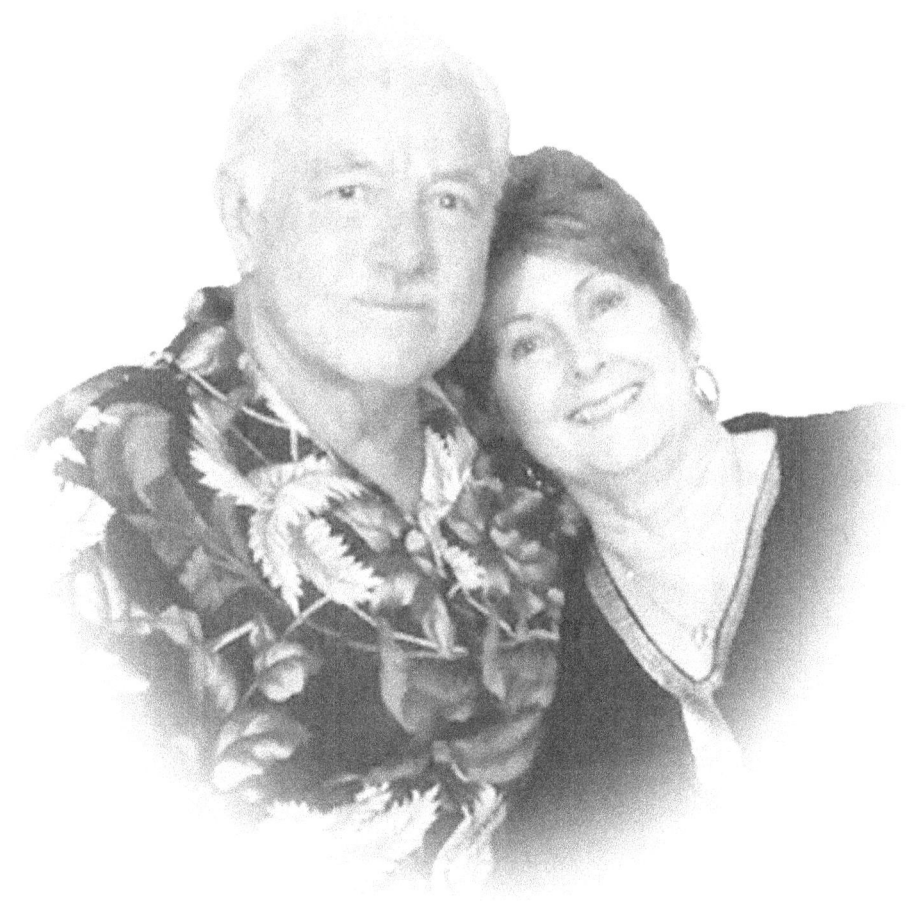

Welcome to
CouchEsthentics®

Many people don't have time or the desire to go to the gym. Many of us won't ever wear spandex, pricey athletic shoes, or work out with high-speed, gut wrenching exercises.

We're tired, lazy, overweight or out of shape, or maybe we think we're just too old. Perhaps the climate keeps us inside or it's not safe to run around the neighborhood we live in. Our video libraries are full of exercise regimens that just plain wore us out or worse, caused us debilitating aches and pains. We've given up on physical fitness and it's causing shortness of breath and sagging muscles. Eventually, this can lead to more physical ailments and even medical emergencies.

Stretching and strengthening your muscles and giving your heart a little workout can be a great way to help achieve a happier, healthier life.

Time, transportation and weather are hurdles for anyone developing and maintaining an adequate workout schedule.

That is why I came up with a simple plan that eliminates the burden of having to put aside time in the day to travel to a gym, dodge the weather to take a walk in the park, or any other obstacle between you and the pursuit of a healthy lifestyle.

You can do it while you are safely at home. Even while you're watching TV!

I call it CouchEsthentics.

Let's be honest, if you're planning to use this book, you're not in tiptop shape, and you're not just a few sit ups away from being fit as a fiddle. That's your business and it's fine with me, but now, in the comfort and privacy of your own home, without the use of any expensive videos, gadgets, or costly equipment, you can work on your strength, flexibility, and overall physical health.

You will be surprised at the changes even a small amount of regular stretching and exercise can make in your daily life.

Please Read This First

If you are currently under a doctor's care, or have been diagnosed with any chronic physical ailments or diseases, it is important to consult your physician before beginning this exercise regimen. In fact, bring in your copy of this book for your doctor to review, just to make sure everything in it is suitable for you.

If you are reading this, you probably didn't run a marathon last weekend or even contemplate running one.

This is a manual for people who often get little or no exercise and that means your body is not ready for heavy workout. However, you can build up your limberness and strength noticeably using these simple techniques.

Some of us have never had an active physical lifestyle. And many, as we go through the pageant of life, slow down, sit more, and in general, eliminate the more strenuous activities of our younger years. That is no reason to stop being fit, and I think that by following these easy exercises, you will be pleased with the progress you will make.

I want you to increase your flexibility, strength, and overall endurance. All of these things are components of good health and can help reduce the risk of a myriad of maladies from heart disease to joint stiffness. Combined with the correct dietary choices and regular participation, I believe that you can feel stronger and more flexible, gain confidence, and become a happier, healthier you.

Please read and follow all the information carefully and remember that it can be very easy to over-exert yourself. Don't try more than the recommended repetitions at the beginning, increasing only after you have done them for at least a couple of weeks or so. Don't worry, that marathon will still be waiting if and when the right time comes.

Please be aware that dizziness or loss of balance might occur when exercising, especially when standing up or looking away from the normal horizon. At the slightest onset, please sit down safely, breathe normally and drink some water.

I highly recommend that you read through this entire book before you begin. If at any time you feel any pain or develop medical conditions that would be exacerbated by any of these exercises, please stop and consult with your doctor before continuing.

You may want to wait three days after your first session to work out again. This will give your body time to grow with the new experience. After that, every other day for a few weeks and then begin a daily routine.

CouchEsthentics®

LET'S WARM UP

Prior to exercising it is important to get the blood flowing throughout the body. This prepares the muscles for action and endurance and helps them to rest and grow afterward.

Remember to drink fluids in order to keep your body and muscles properly hydrated. Nothing works better than good old water. Avoid carbonated, sugary, or caffeinated energy products.

WALK IN PLACE

If you are watching television, the opening credits or commercials, are a perfect time to start walking in place.

1. Start with a three-minute walk.

2. Let your arms slightly swing gently at your side, lifting up your forearms to swing back and forth.

3. As you progress, and feel comfortable with this, increase the duration and speed along with raising your knees a little higher.

This will increase your overall blood flow and get your body ready to perform all the other exercises.

Always rest for a short period before continuing and drink some water.

If at any time you feel weak or light headed, please sit down and breathe normally.

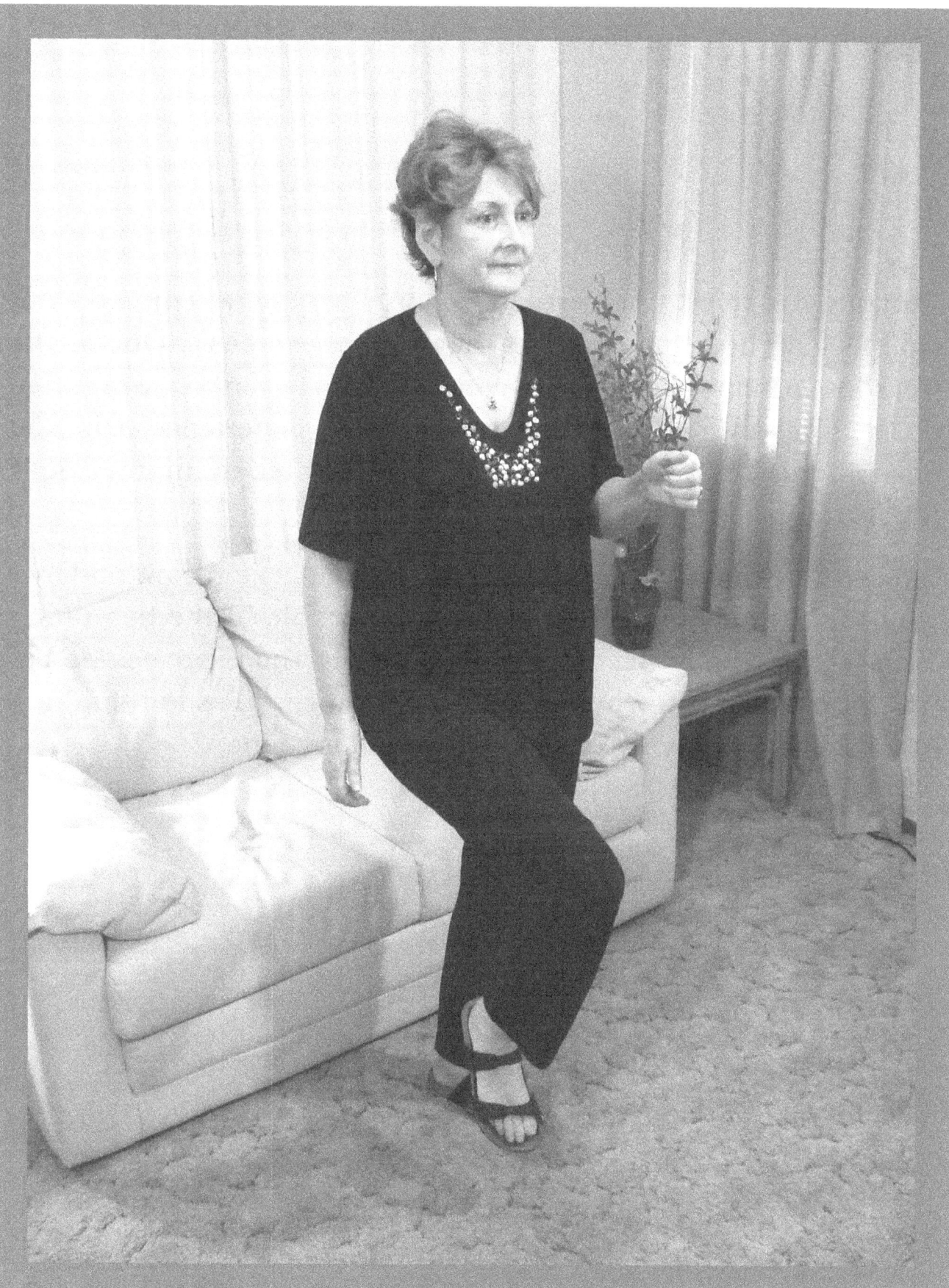

Anything marked **"Advanced"** should **NOT** be attempted until you feel comfortable doing all the original exercises. One of the reasons so many people fail to continue with any exercise regimen is that they overexert themselves early on, experience pain and lose interest. You have the rest of your new life to improve, let's make it work for you!

Please note that all the photographs show full extensions and that you should only extend as far as comfortable in the beginning and let your body become accustomed to the exercises before pushing yourself further. Don't do too much, too soon thinking it all seems so easy. Pace yourself and be patient.

NOW LET'S STRETCH A LITTLE

Almost all of these exercises can be done sitting on the edge of your seat or standing. Find your own comfort zone and increase repetitions and duration only when you are ready.

Remember to visualize what you are trying to achieve with each exercise. When stretching, see yourself extending. Focus your body on the task at hand, relax and let the tension in your muscles escape.

FINGER STRETCH

1. Stretch both arms in front of you and spread your fingers as wide as comfortable.

2. Slowly bring your arms out to the sides.

3. Wriggle your outspread fingers and then return your hands to the front.

4. Bring your hands down to your sides. Rest and repeat.

Repeat three times to start off and increase to 10 repetitions after a few weeks.

FINGER FLEX

I call this the "Spider on a mirror."

1. Place your hands together with fingers spread and elbows out, but slightly lowered.

2. Raise your elbows and slowly push your hands apart keeping only the finger tips in contact.

3. Then press your hands back together until your palms are touching. Remember to lower your elbows enough to avoid discomfort.

Repeat three times. Increase to 10 times after a few weeks.

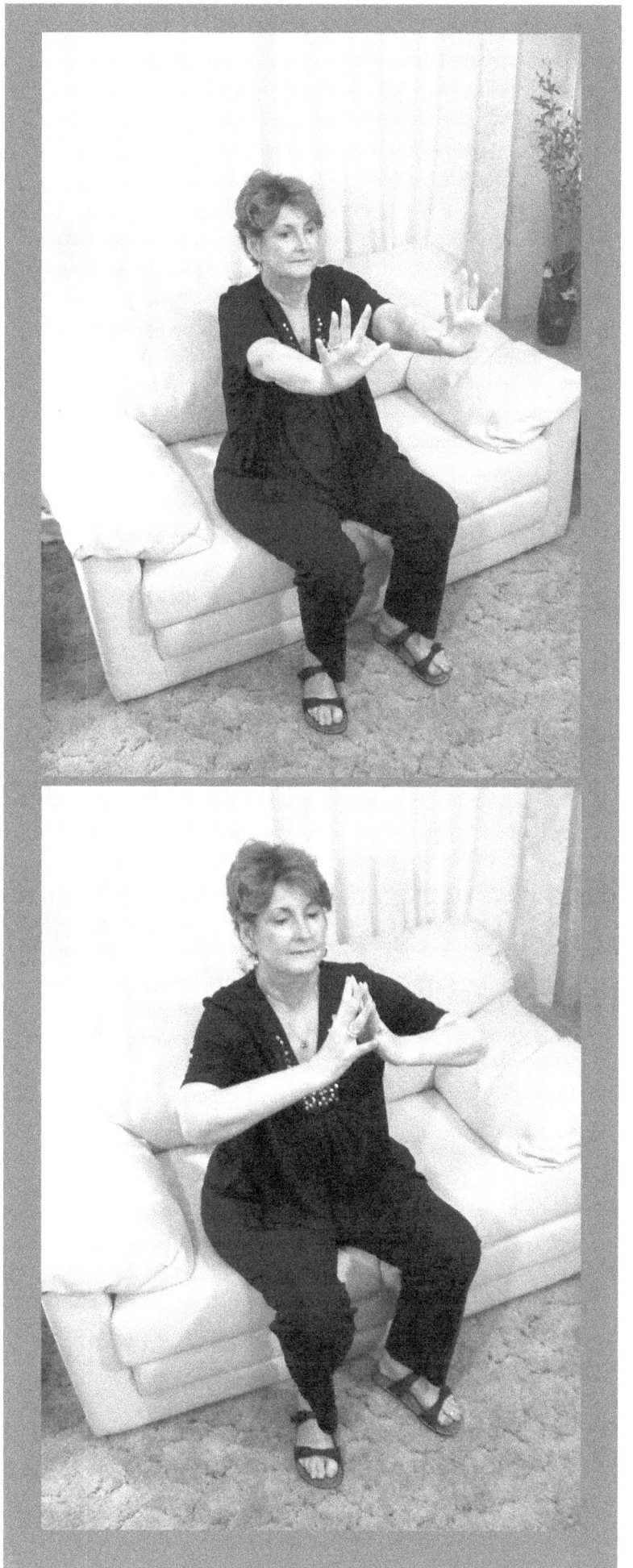

REVERSE FINGER STRETCH

1. Sit with fingers interlocked and raise elbows to chest level.

2. Slowly push hands out, stretching fingers.

Hold for a count of three and return hands to starting position and relax. Increase pressure and time held in position as limberness grows.

Remember to start your regimen slowly. It all seems simple, but weak muscles need work at first and you have plenty of time to better yourself.

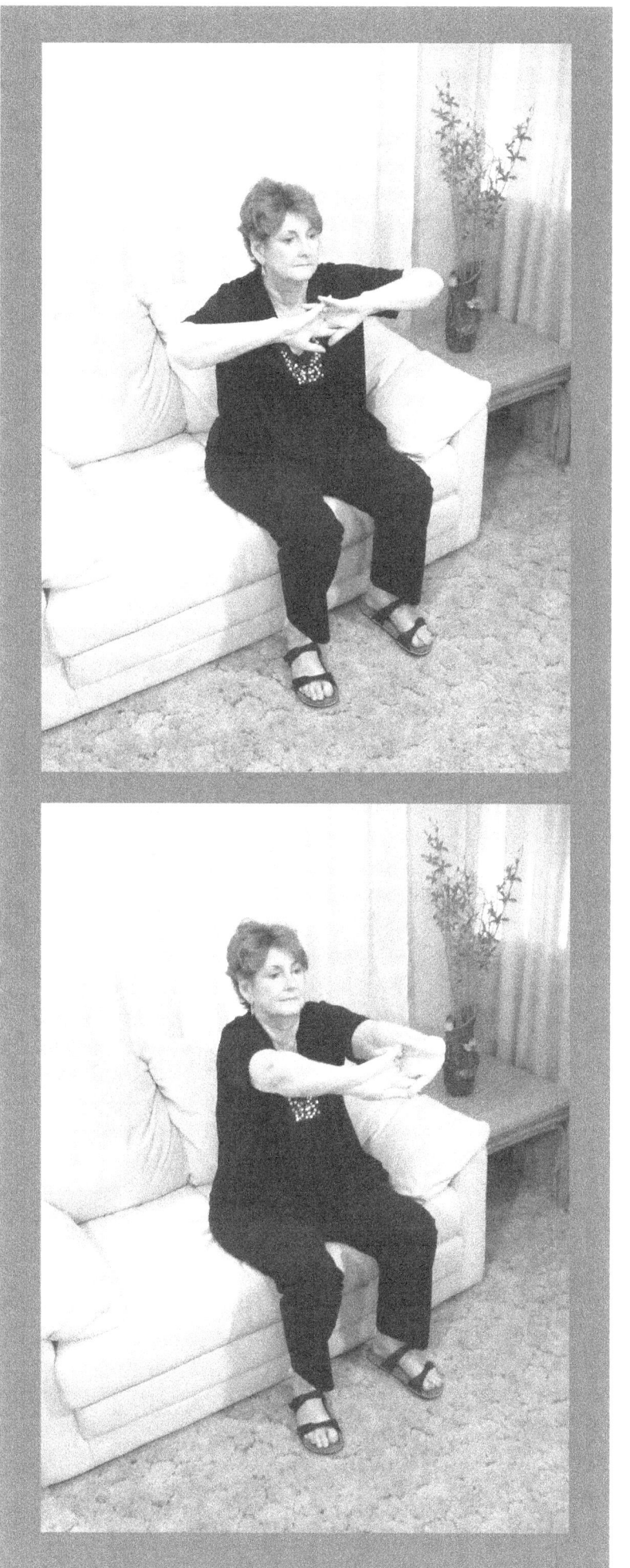

WRIST FLEX

1. Stretch your arms in front of you with your fingers pointed out.

2. Rotate your hands in small circles, moving them in opposite directions. Start with 10 seconds and eventually work up to 20 seconds.

Reverse direction for another 10 to 20 seconds to make sure all the muscles get equal work.

As you feel more limber, enlarge the circles and spread your fingers.

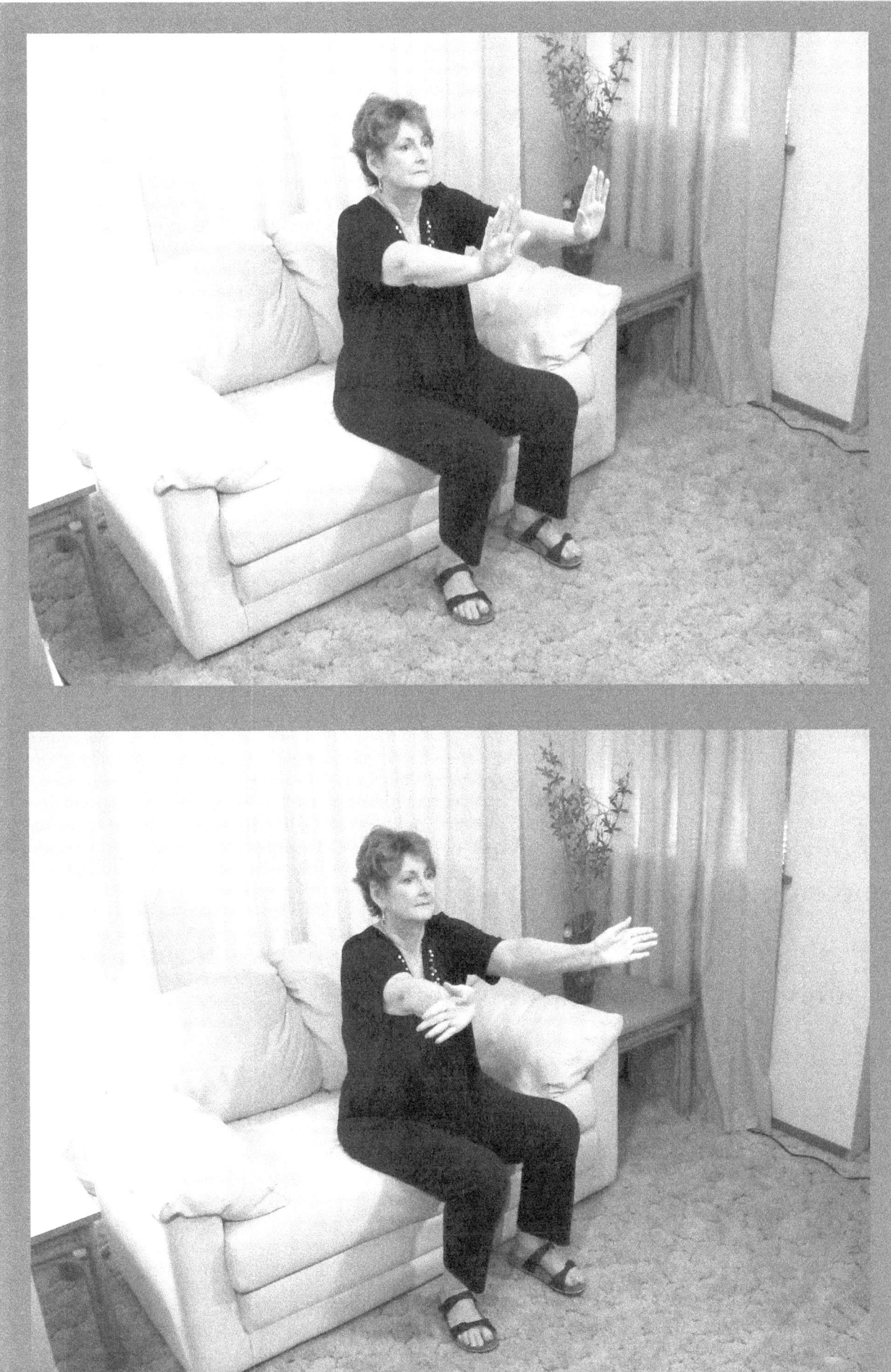

REVERSE FINGER PRESS

1. Bend your right arm inward with palm facing downward and fingers pointing toward the floor.

2. Place your left hand against the backs of your fingers, and while applying slight pressure, raise your fingers up to flat.

3. Using your palm to apply pressure once more, lower your fingers, resisting the force.

Repeat three times. Switch hands and do the same with your left hand.

PART TWO

1. Now with the fingers of your right hand pointed upward, place your left hand against the fingers of your right.

2. Push your right hand back, resisting slightly. Return to a flat position, all the while resisting slightly.

Switch hands after three repetitions.

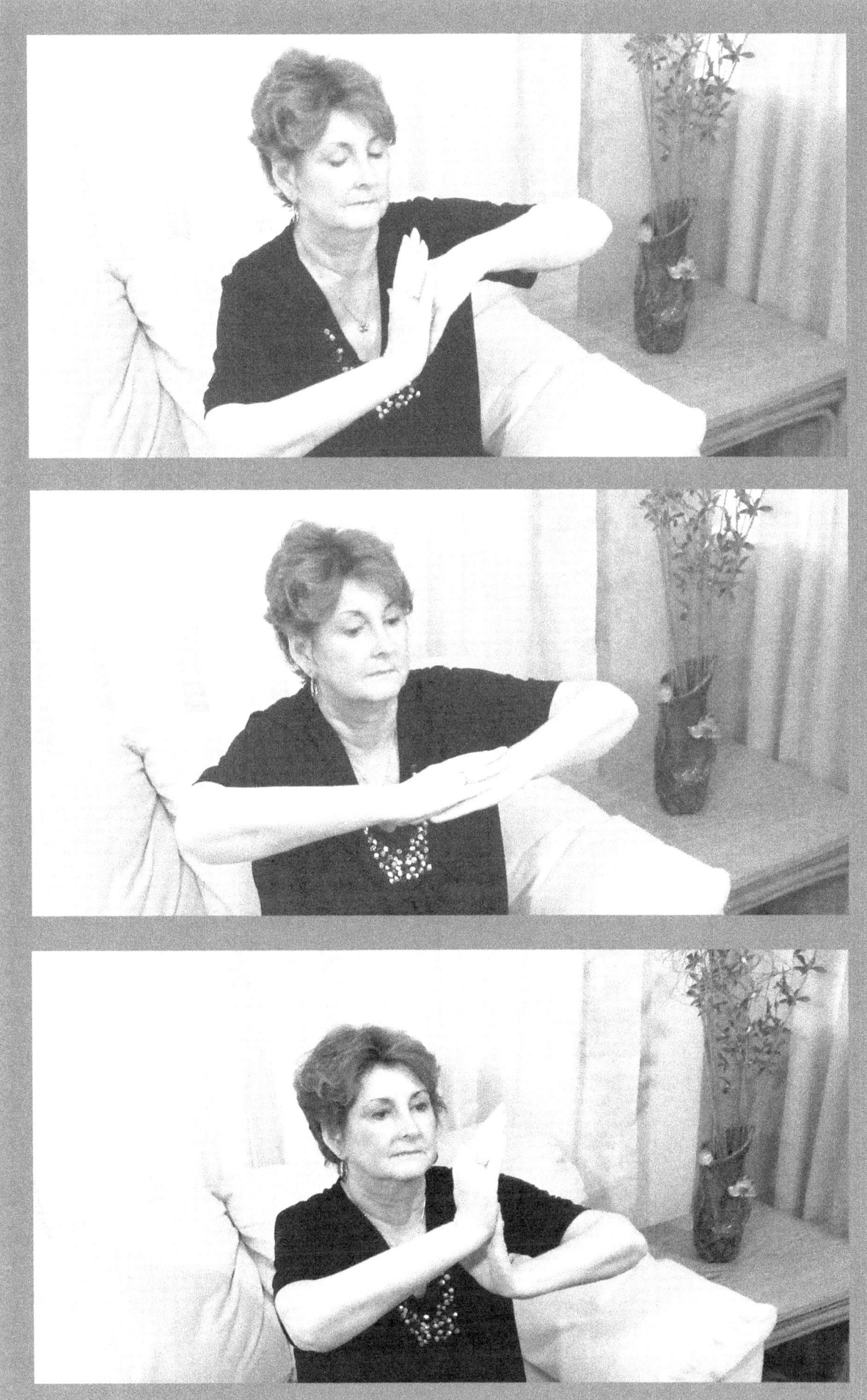

ARM ROTATION

This is best done standing, but can also be done sitting with smaller rotations.

1. Hold your hands out to the side and slowly rotate your arms in small circles, increasing the size of the circles as you go.

Don't windmill! Go slowly.

2. Continue for five to 10 seconds, and then reverse direction.

3. Slowly make smaller circles until you have returned to the starting position.

Increase size of circles and length of time to 15 to 30 seconds as time goes by.

Try one complete cycle, small circles to big and then back to small. When you feel comfortable with that, add a another cycle.

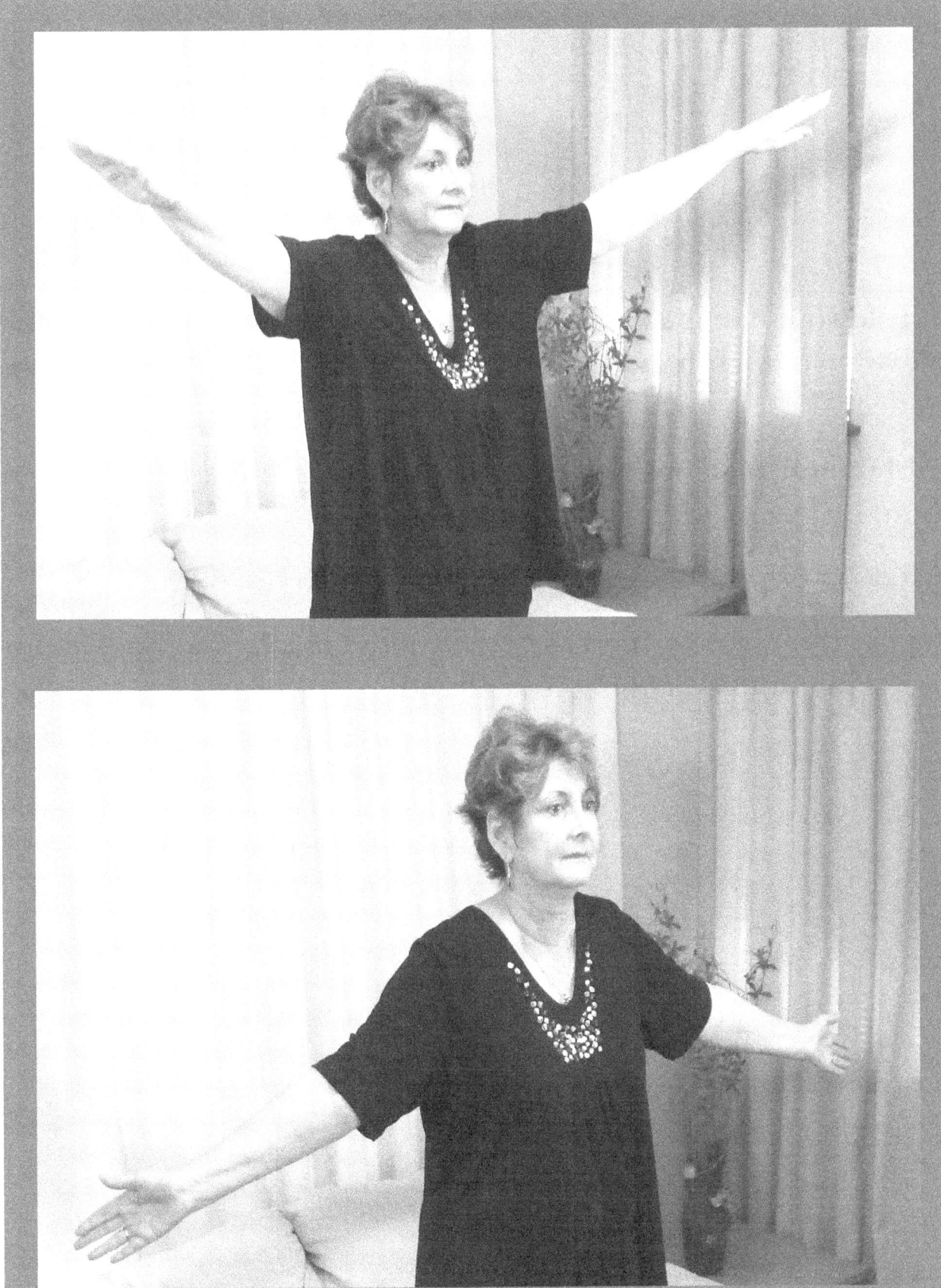

ARM STRETCH

1. Hold your hands near your shoulders, reach up and out to your left with your left hand as far as you can stretch in a comfortable mode.

2. Maintain that position with your fingers outstretched for a count of five.

3. Return to starting position and then reach out to the right.

Repeat three times. Increase repetitions, reach, and time spent stretching until a 10 count is achieved.

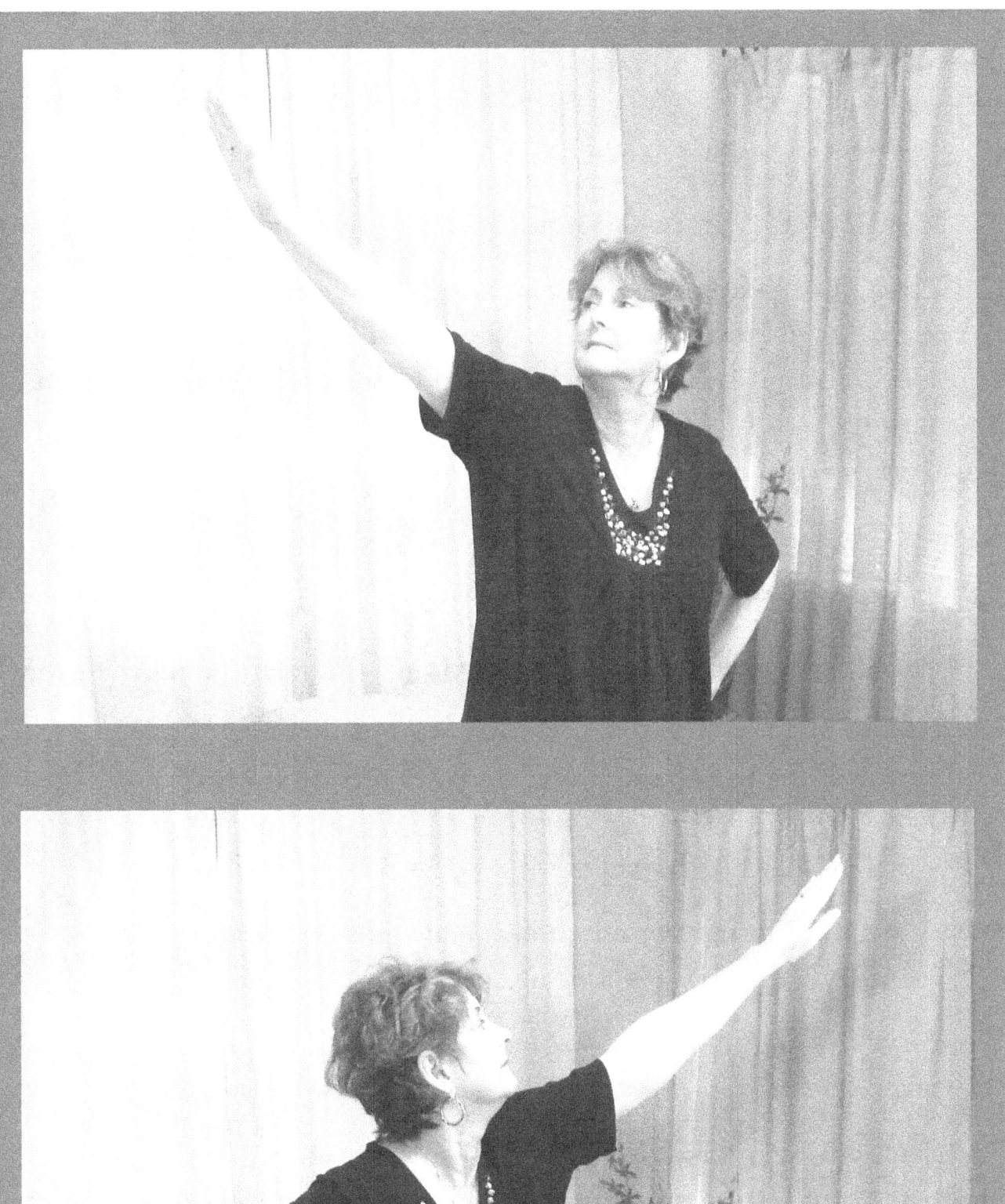

OVERHEAD ARM STRETCH

1. Stand, with arms at your side.

2. Reach your left arm up and stretch it over the top of your head as far as comfortable and stretch as if you were reaching for something towards the right. Slightly bend your torso in that direction.

Hold for a count of three, then slowly extend your arm straight up, and bring it back down to your side.

Repeat three times on both sides.

Increase repetitions and depth of your bend as you become more limber.

Remember to stretch slowly and avoid over reaching.

ADVANCED OVERHEAD STRETCH

Do not attempt advanced exercises until you feel comfortable and at ease with the others.

1. Reach your left hand as close to straight over your head as comfortable.

2. Grab your fingers with your right hand and pull softly, leaning with the pull. Take your arm as far as comfortable and hold for three seconds. Repeat using right hand.

3. Do three repetitions to start. Once you notice improvement, try to pull hand farther over your head and increase hold time.

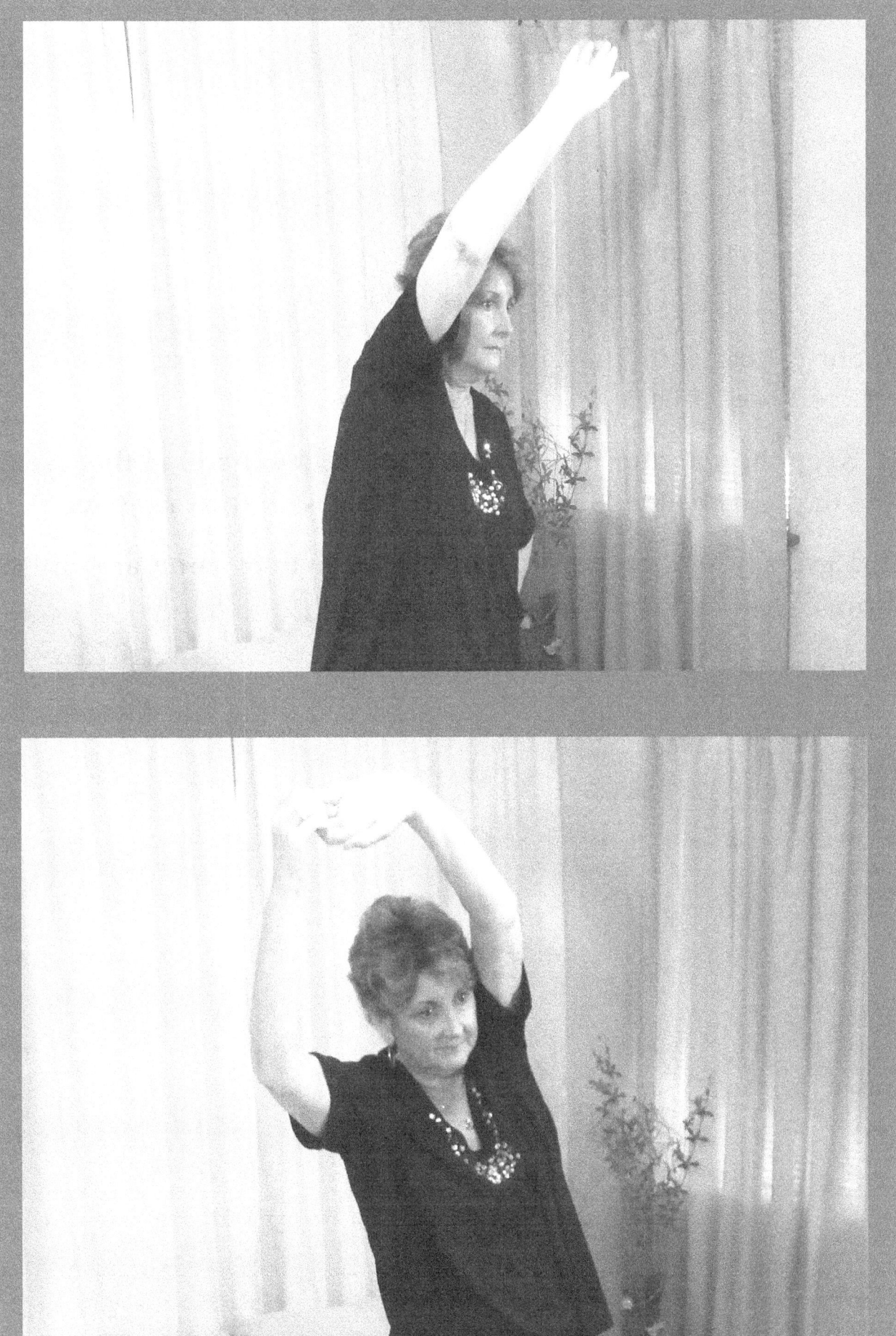

SHOULDER ROTATION

1. Shrug your shoulders and move them in a forward rotation for five to 10 seconds.

2. Keep the rotations small at first, and then increase the size as the days go by and you feel comfortable with the movement.

3. Reverse the direction of your rotations for same amount of time.

Increase to 15 seconds as you progress.

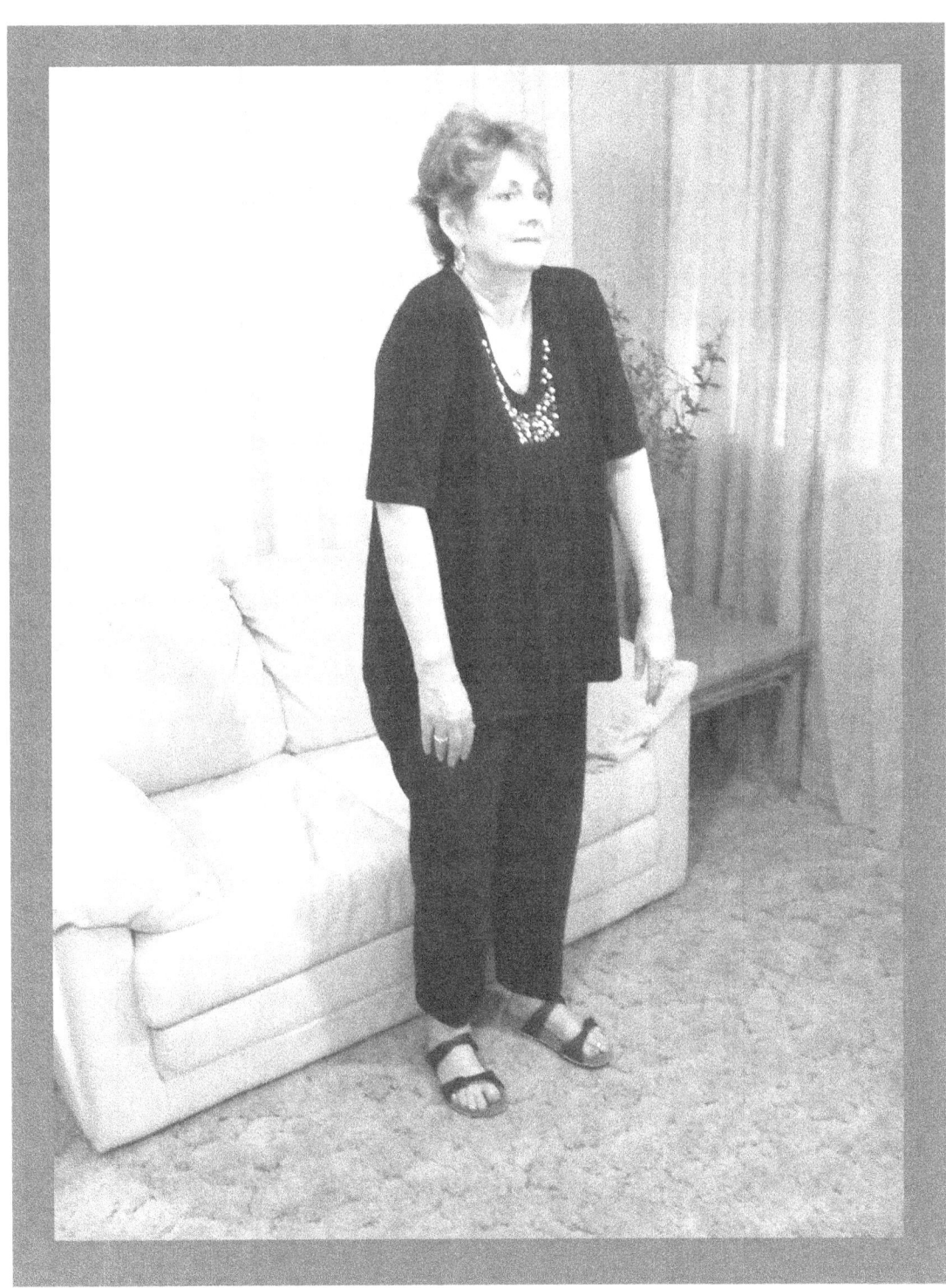

ANKLE AND FOOT ROTATION

1. Sit at the edge of your seat with feet flat on the floor. Extend one leg as far as comfortable so your foot is slightly off the floor.

2. Slowly rotate your foot, keeping your leg outstretched. Reverse direction and finish by pointing your toes away from you and wiggling them.

3. With your leg still straight, slowly try to point your toes back at you, stretching the tendon at the back of your heel as comfortably as possible. Hold for a three count and then place your foot back on the floor.

4. Repeat with the other foot.

Do three repetitions to start and then increase number of rotations.

Remember, do not overdo this as you will feel your tendons stretching and the health of your tendons and muscles are very important to your walking ability.

Always remember not to make jerky movements and just apply pressure in a soft, but constant level. This will allow you to gauge your abilities and not cause any discomfort or injury.

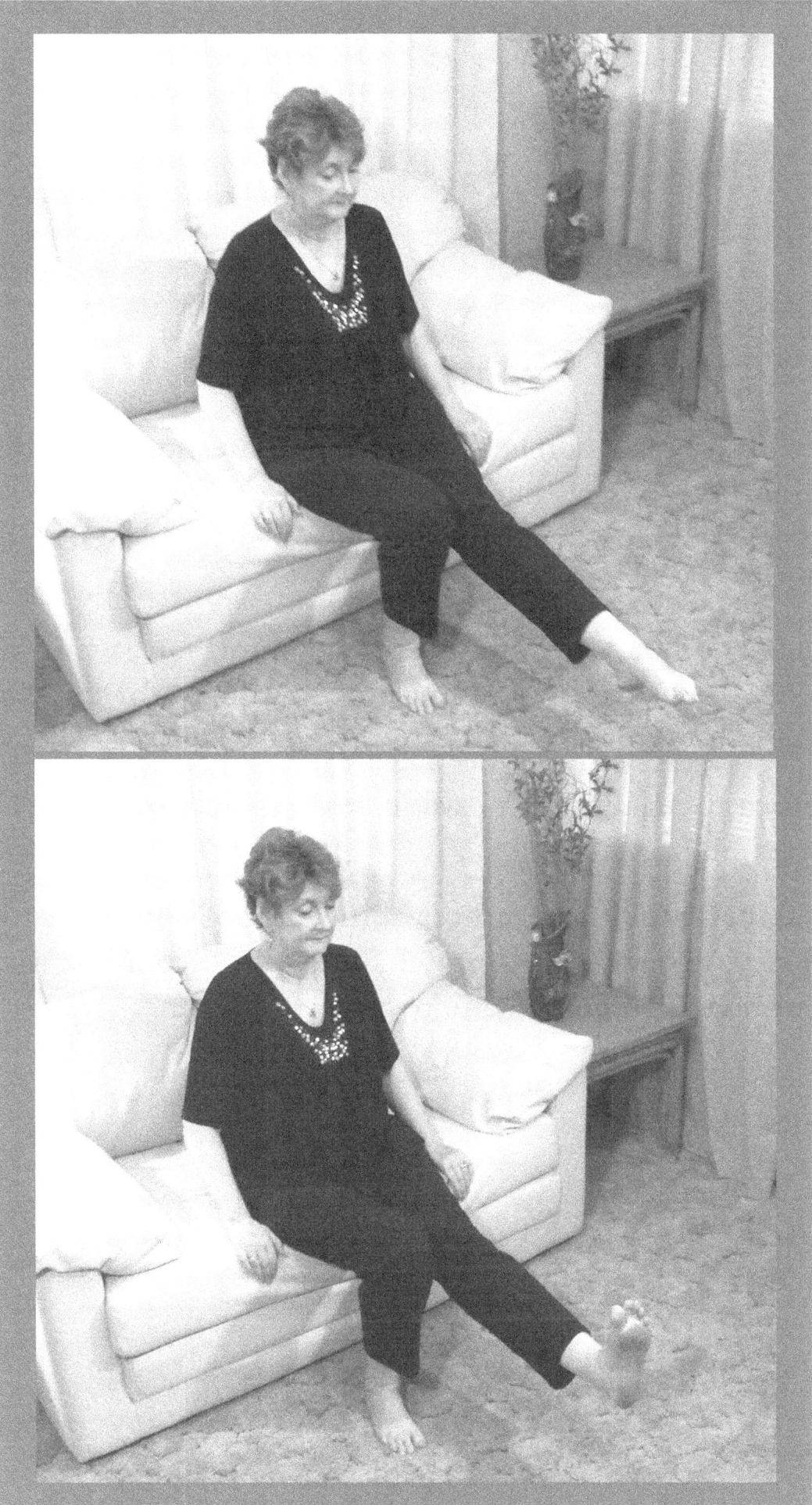

FORWARD BEND

1. Sit with your feet spread a little wider than shoulder width, toes pointing upward and knees straight. Lean forward slowly with your arms hanging between your legs. **DO NOT BOB UP AND DOWN!**

2. Relax and bend forward as far as comfortable, while keeping your knees locked in a straight position. Hold for three counts, breathing normally.

3. Return to an upright position and repeat three times with a short rest in between.

You might feel a little tightness at the back of your knees and the small of your back as you stretch, but you will increase the depth of your bend and become more limber over time.

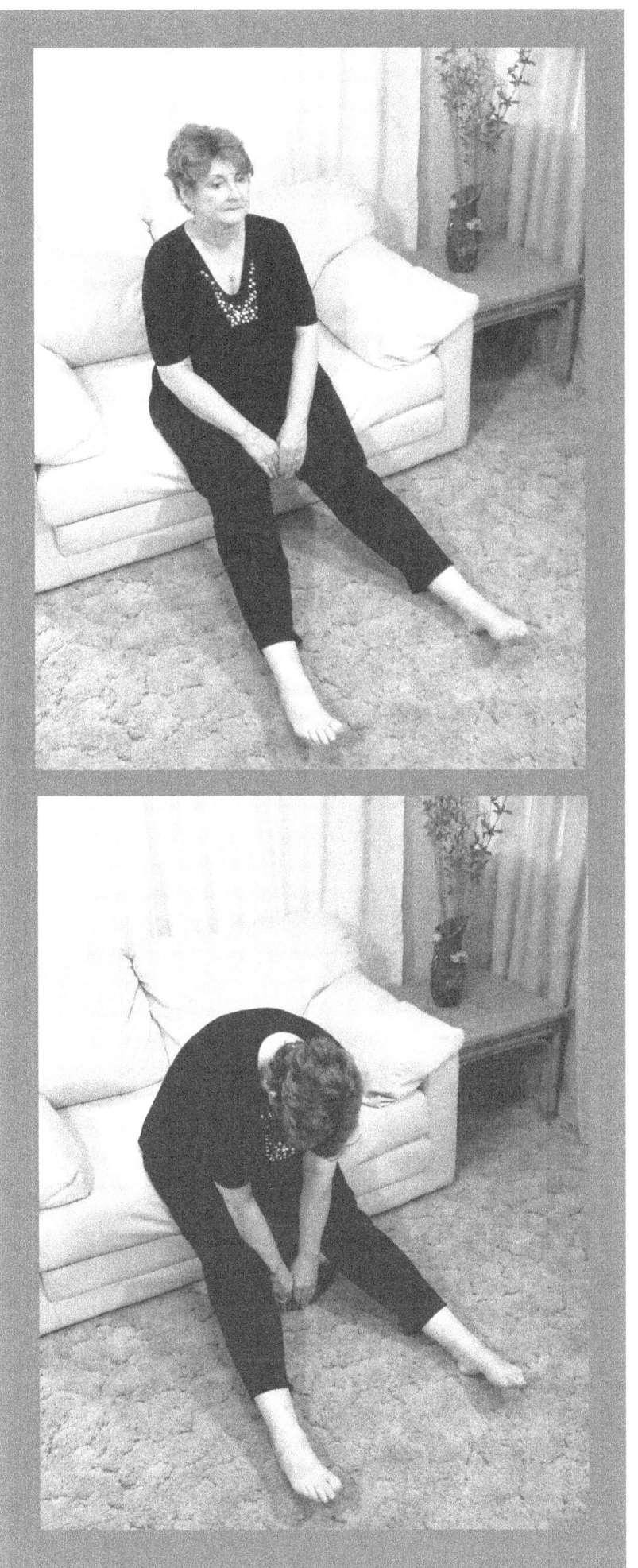

ADVANCED FORWARD BEND

Once you have achieved greater flexibility and a deeper stretch:

1. Keep your feet together and bring your hands down, lightly grasping your legs. Hold for a count of five.

2. Pull tighter on your legs and work up to holding for a count of 10. After you see some real progress in your flexibility and endurance, increase up to a count of 20.

1. Move up to a standing position. With feet spread about shoulder width apart, allow your hands to hang down in front of you and bend at the waist. Dangle for a count of three to start and return to an upright position. Increase distance and length of time as you feel comfortable.

IF you have any trouble balancing, or feel any dizziness, please stop immediately and sit down, breathing normally.

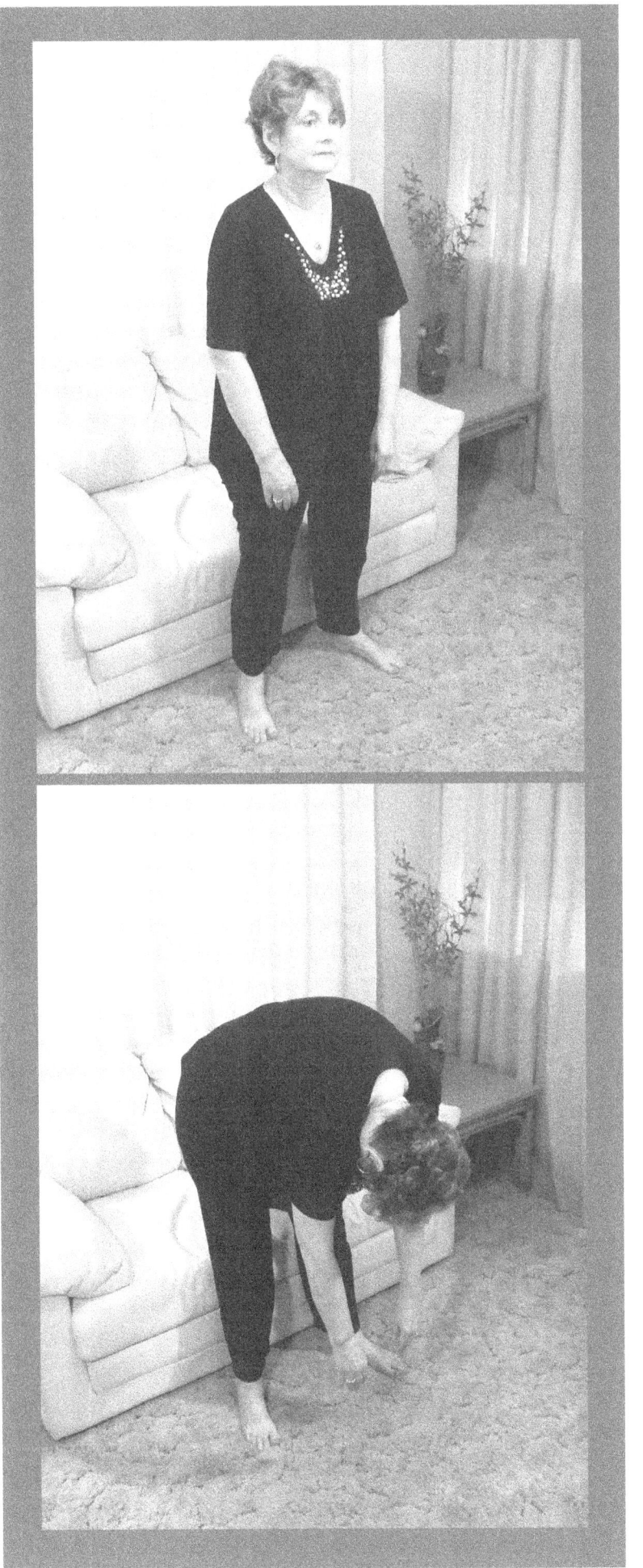

TORSO TWIST

1. Sit or stand and place your hands as close to your shoulders as possible with elbows pointing out to your sides.

2. Slowly turn your head and torso to the left as far as comfortable. Hold that position for a count of three and return to start.

Repeat three times on both sides.

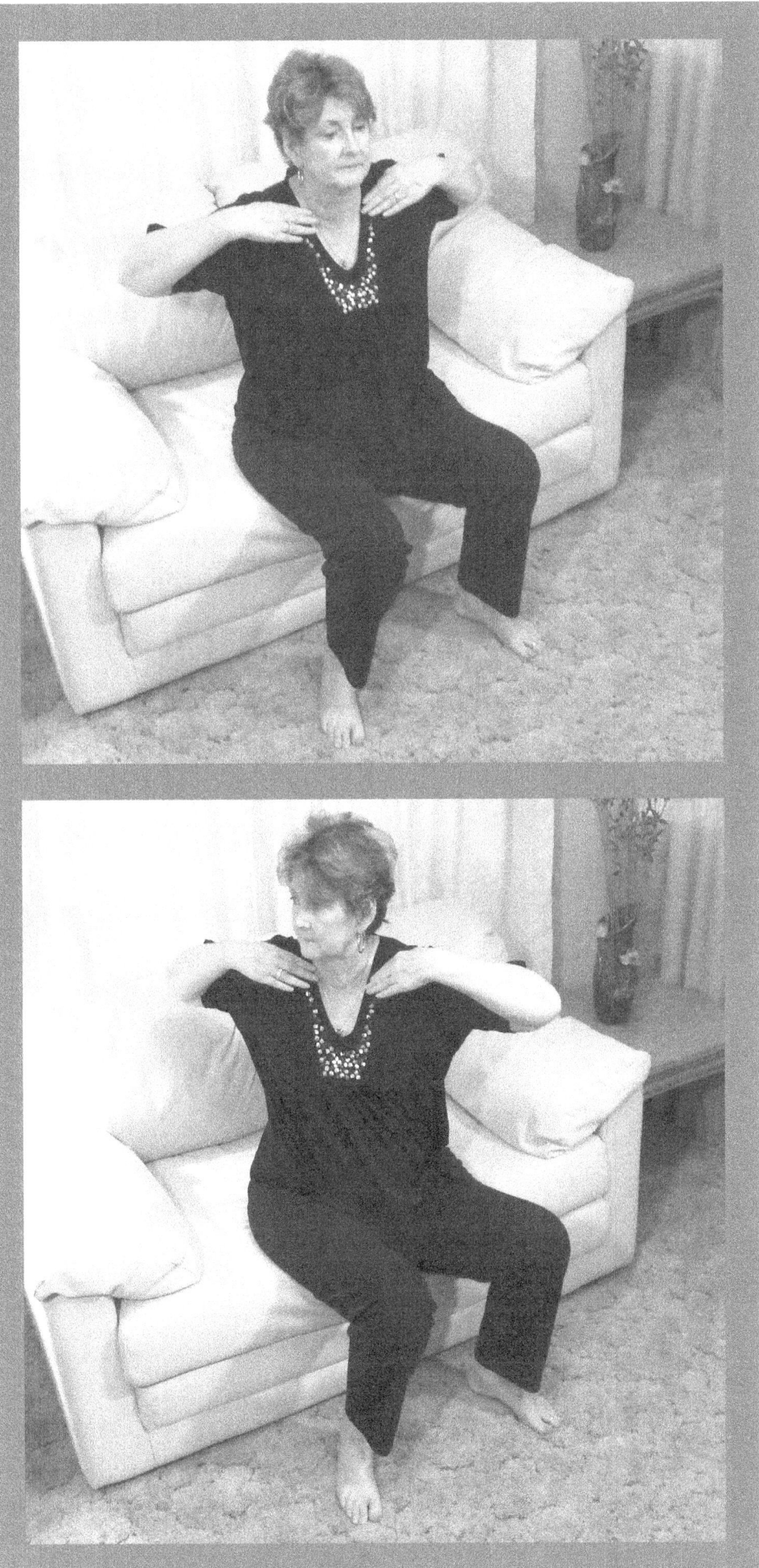

TORSO ROTATION

1. Stand or sit at front of your seat with your feet slightly wider than shoulder width apart and your hands on your waist.

2. Lean forward slightly and circle your entire torso to the right three times.

Repeat to the left, eventually increasing the depth and number of rotations to a maximum of 10.

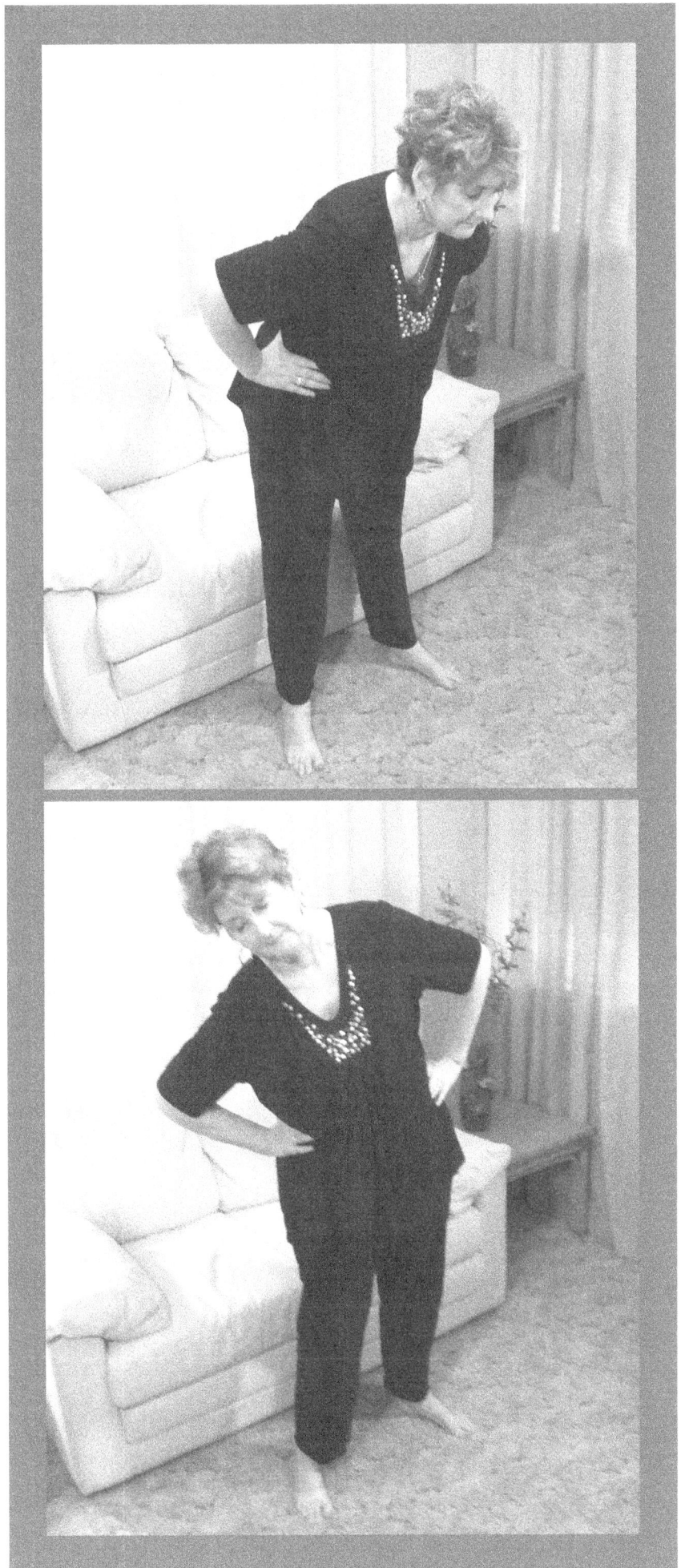

TORSO STRETCH

1. Place your hands up toward your ears with elbows facing out.

2. Lean upper torso to the left and hold for a count of three.

3. Return to an upright position and lean to the right, holding for three counts again, breathing normally.

Repeat three times for each side. Increase depth and repetitions when you can.

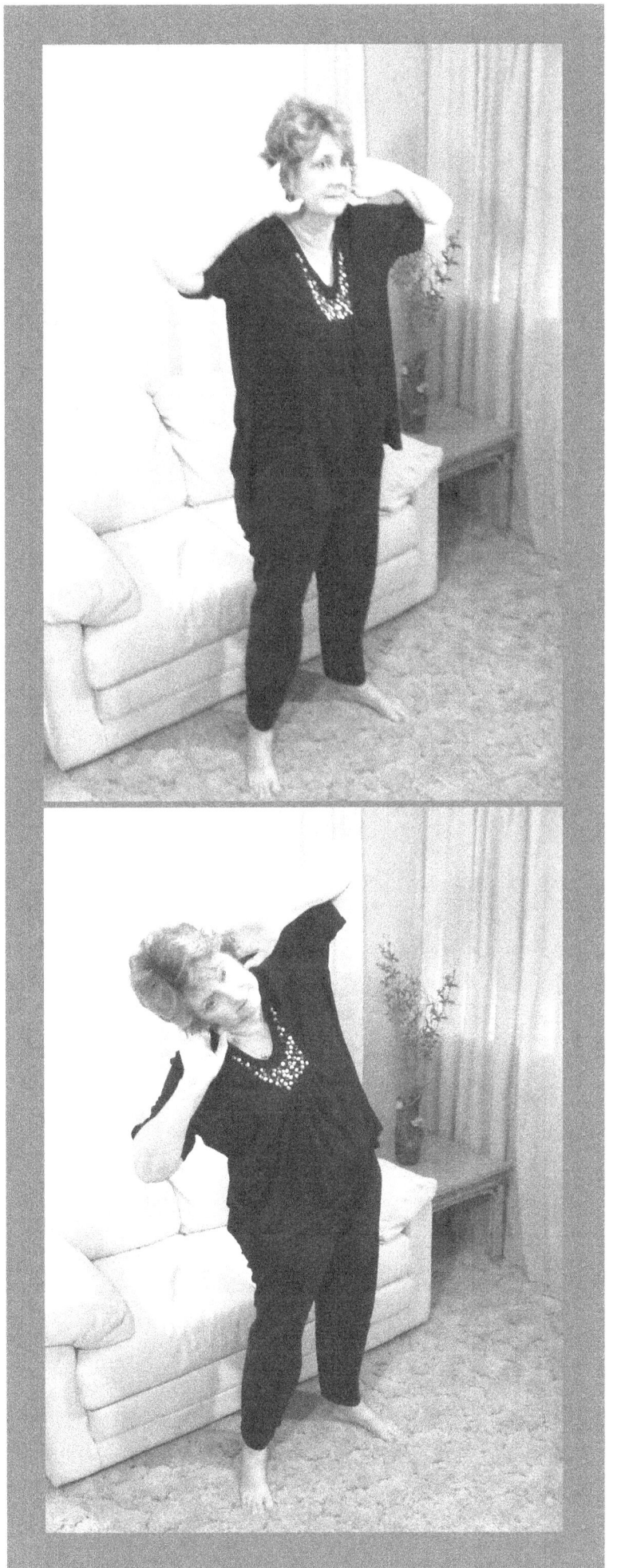

CROSS ARM STRETCH

1. Stand or sit with your feet shoulder width apart. Take your right hand and slowly reach across your body toward the opposite shoulder, looking in that direction and keeping your shoulders forward. Remember to go only as far as your body says is comfortable.

Hold for a count of three.

2. Reach in the other direction with the left hand.

Repeat this three times for each hand, slowly increasing to 10.

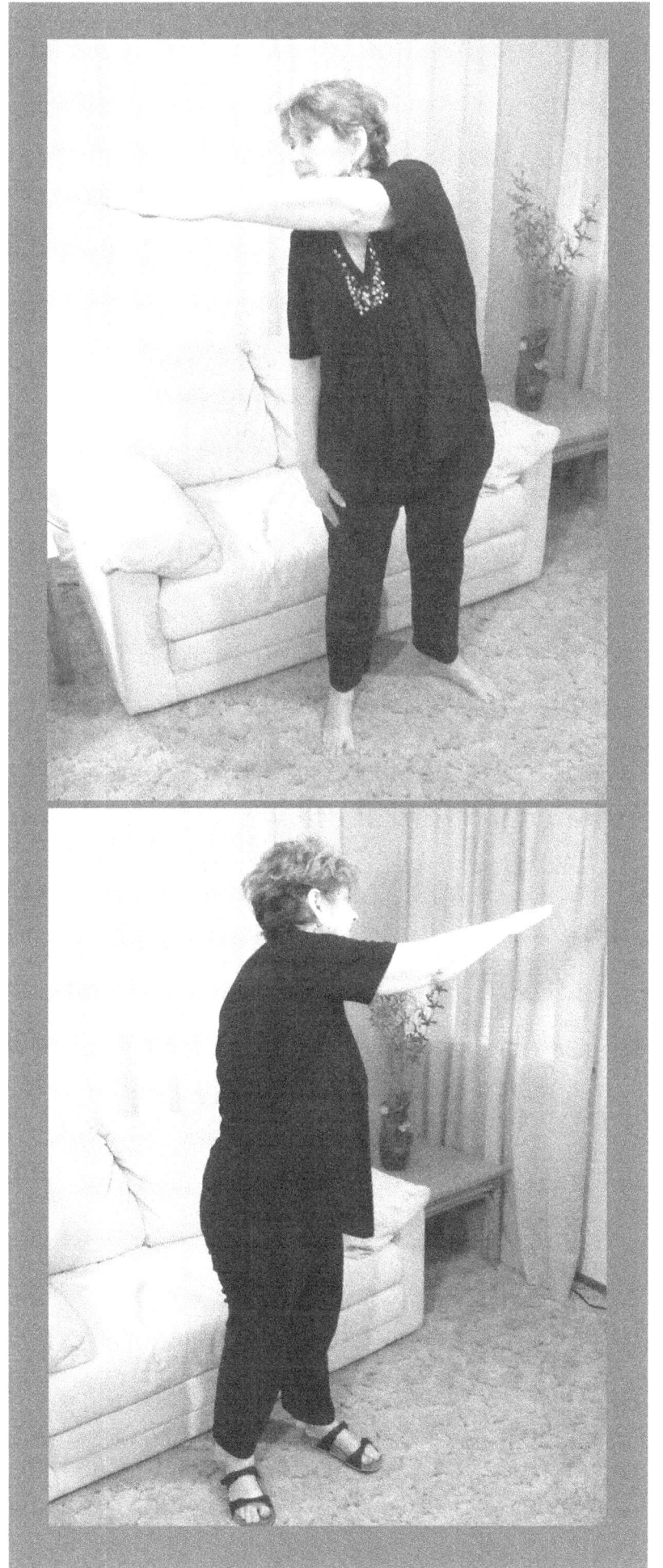

CHICKEN WING

1.   Make fists and bring them up as close to your armpits as comfortable, with elbows out.

2. Pull your elbows back slowly, keeping your fists near your armpits.

3. Hold for a count of three and then return. Increase repetitions and speed as you improve in flexibility.

4. As you advance, repeat steps one and two, but rotate your elbows in a circular motion all the while keeping your fists in the same position. Reverse direction after five rotations.

It is not uncommon to hear some cracking sounds from your shoulders when you start.

Remember to perform these exercises at your own ability level.

Clucking noises are optional.

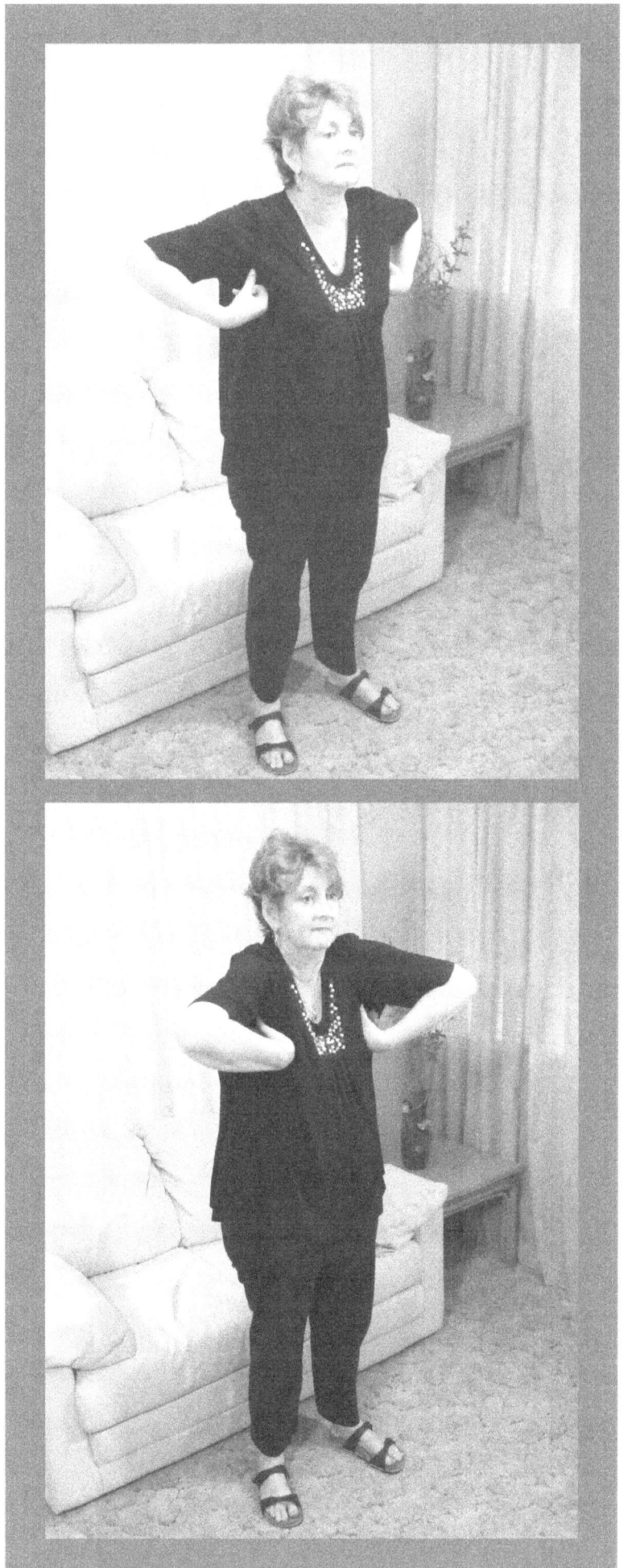

NECK STRETCH

1. Sit with your head facing forward, turn your head to the right as far as comfortable and hold for a three count.

2. Turn your head to the left as far as comfortable and hold for a three count.

3. Face forward and tilt your head back and hold for a three count.

4. Now let your head slowly drop straight forward and hold for a three count.

Repeat this three times.

As you grow more limber, you will notice that you can turn your head farther and hold for a slightly longer time.

Remember not to snap your head in any direction and recognize your limitations.

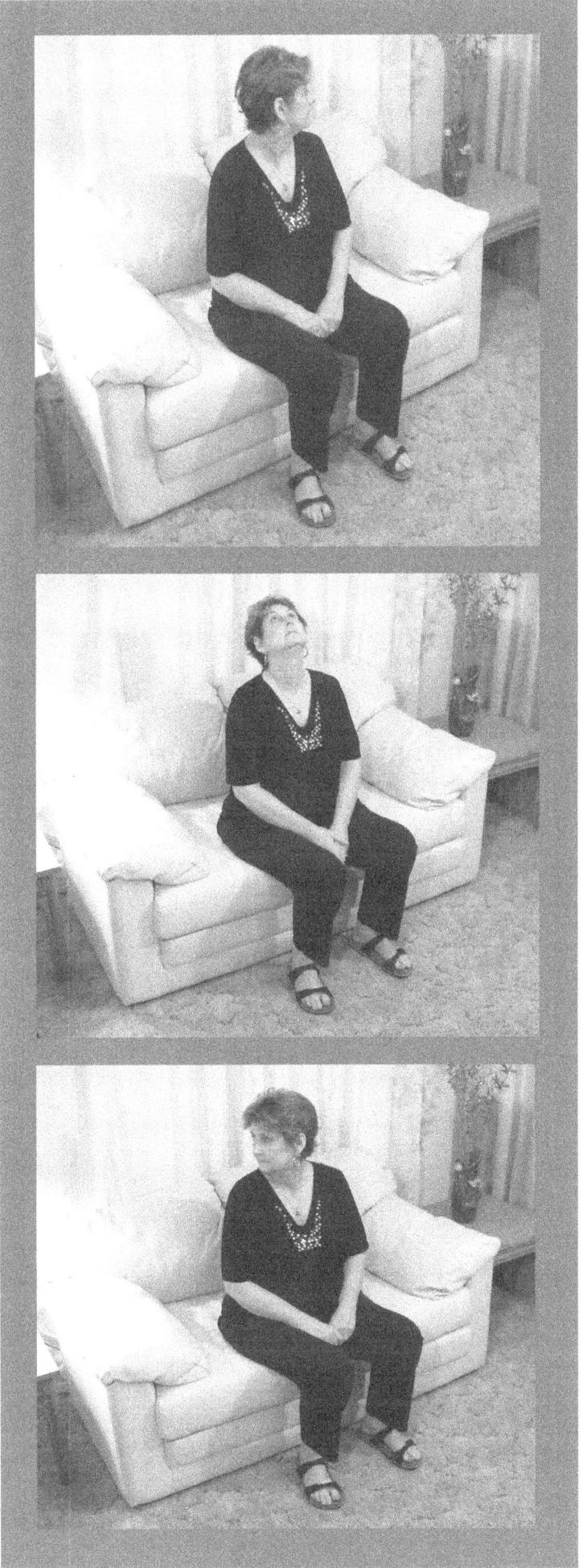

NECK ROTATION

1. Sit with your hands on your hips. Lean your head forward and try to place your chin on your chest.

2. Slowly roll your head to the left. Gently continue around to the back and right side, until you have completed a full rotation.

3. Do three rotations and rest. Then rotate in the opposite direction.

Be gentle when stretching your neck. Don't force any movement.

It is possible your neck will make some noise while doing this so don't be alarmed.

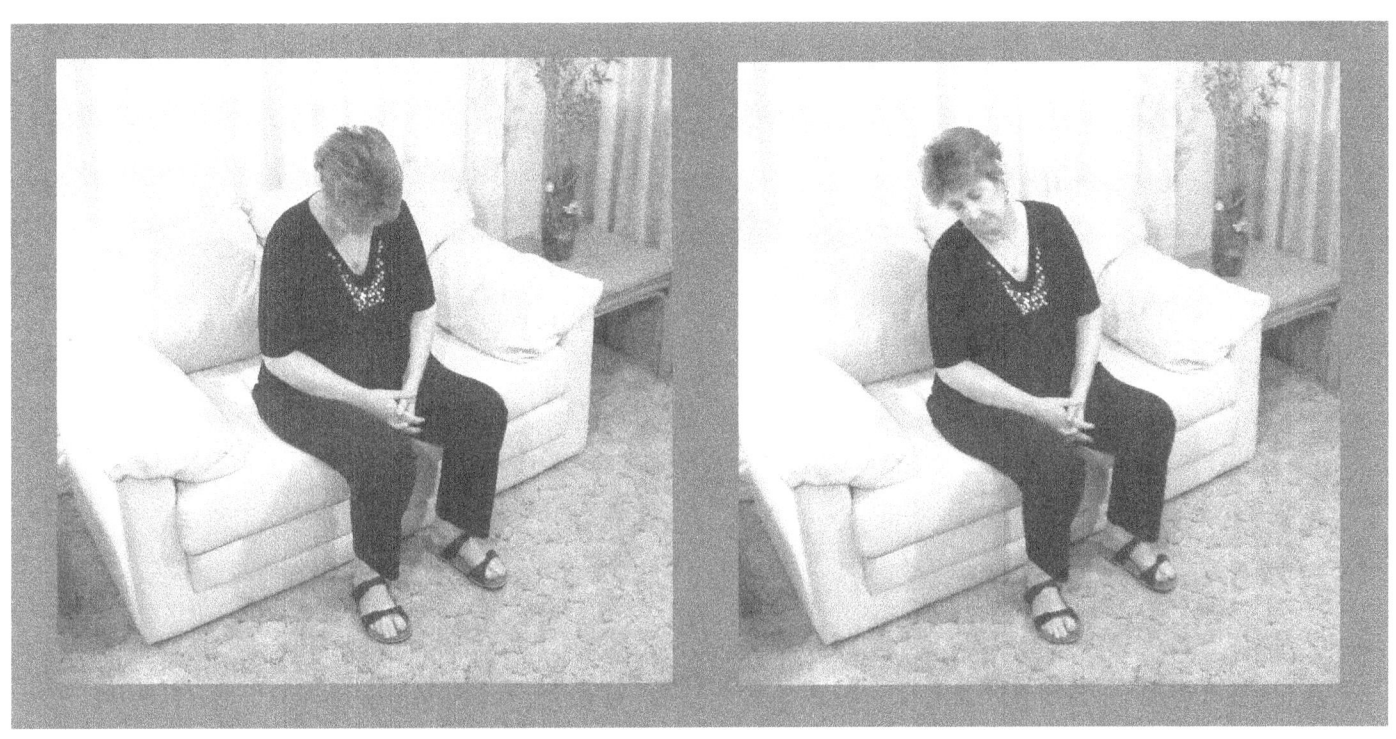

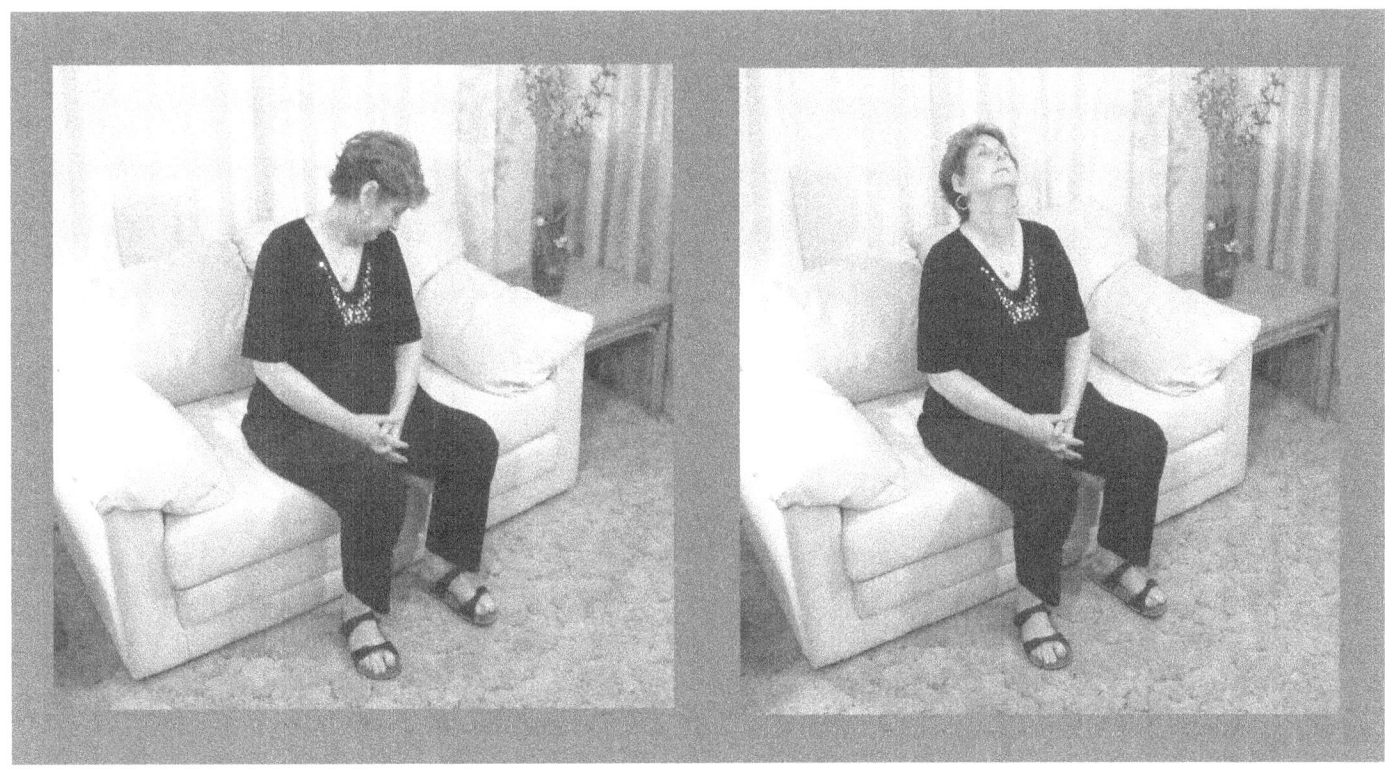

BACK ARCH

1. Sit on the edge of the couch, holding your arms above your head.

2. Look up at your arms and bend your back slightly. Hold for a count of three.

Repeat three times.

This gentle exercise is intended to lightly stretch your muscles and limber up your spine.

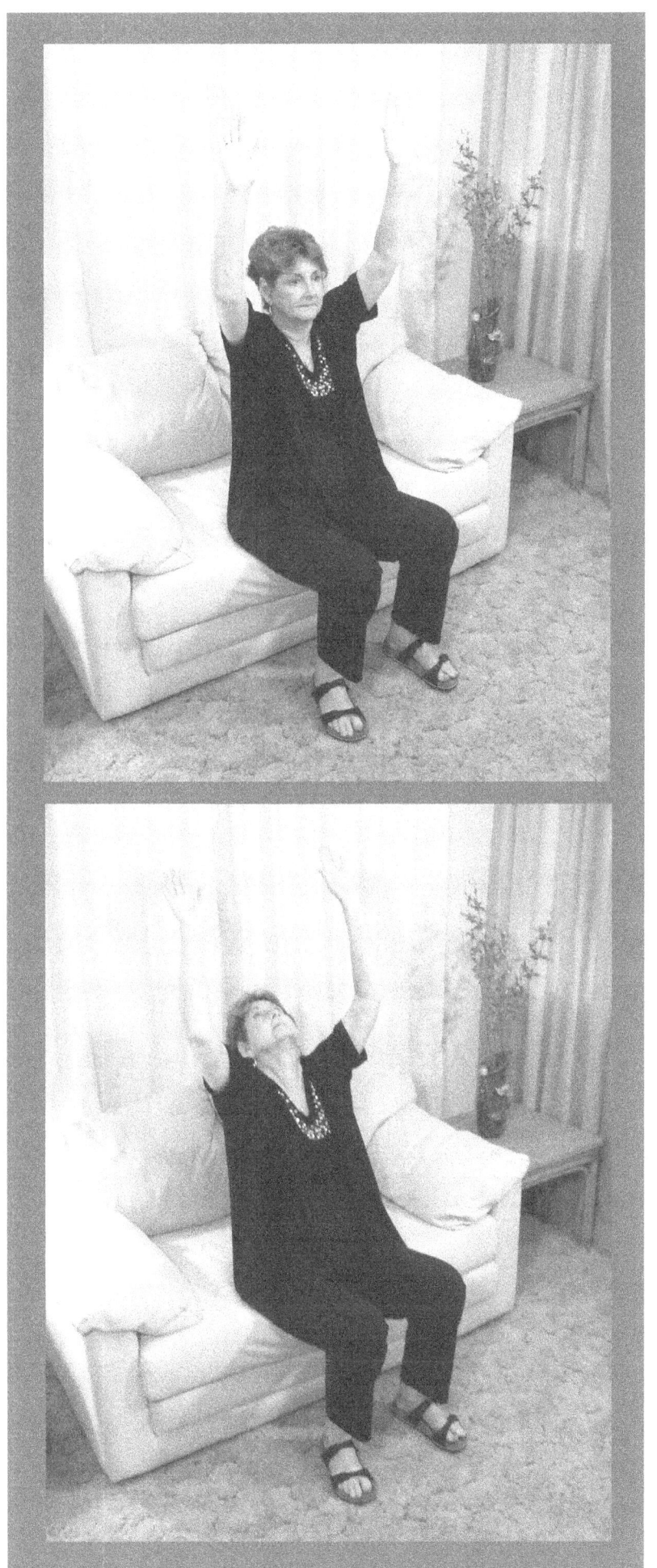

GROIN STRETCH

1. Sit on the front of the couch with your feet shoulder width apart.

2. Clasp your knees from the top with your fingers inside of each knee.

3. Keep your feet in place and slowly spread your knees by pulling with your hands. Your feet will start to roll to the side.

4. Pull until you reach a comfortable limit and then hold for a count of three.

5. Close your knees, applying resistance with your hands.

Repeat three times, increasing the width of your foot stance, repetitions, and time held as your muscles stretch and grow.

Please go easy at first. A pulled groin muscle can be painful and would take some time to heal. You have the rest of your new life to make this work for you, so once again, please don't push yourself beyond your capacity.

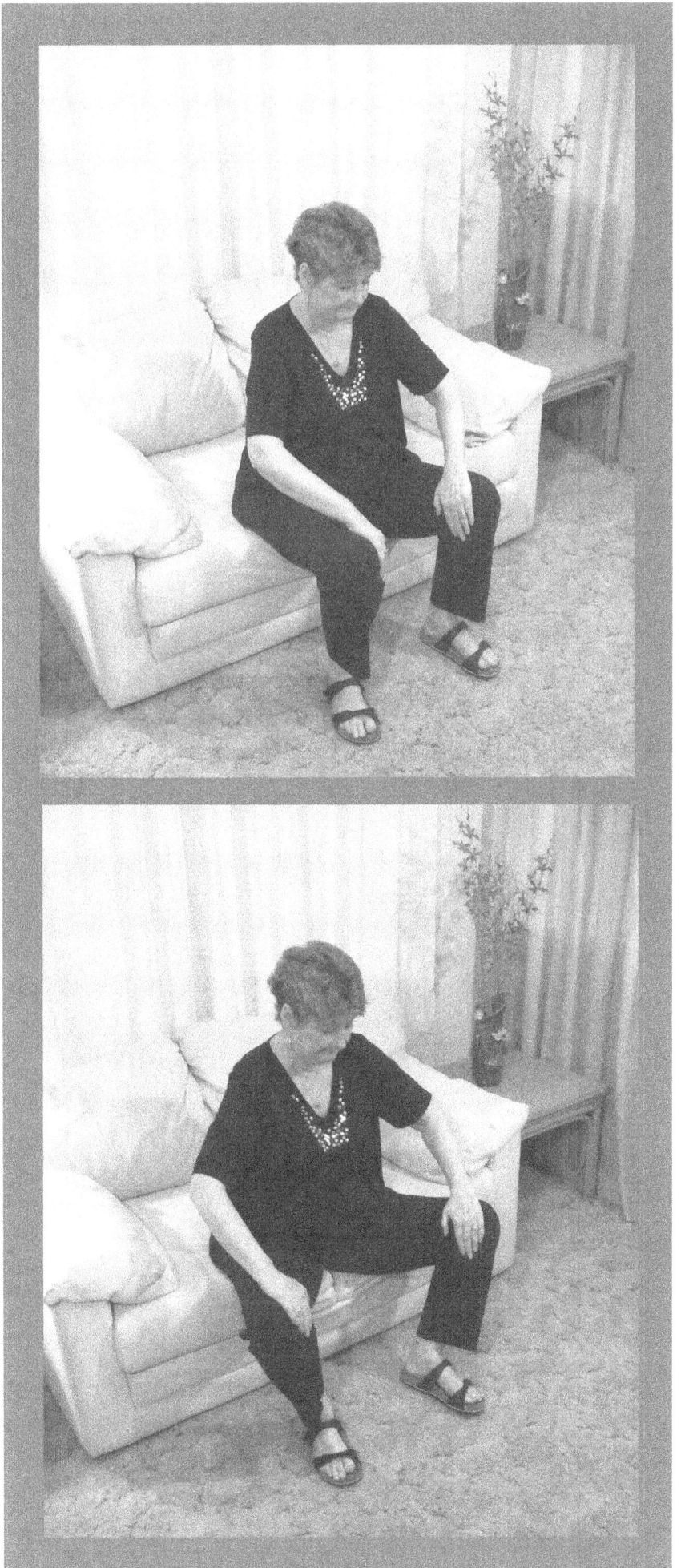

JACK KNIFE

1. Sit on the edge of the couch, with both feet stretched straight out in front of you.

2. Bring one knee up toward you and try to grasp it with both hands.

3. Pull your knee in as close to you as you can and hold for a count of three.

Repeat with other knee. Do this twice with each knee, slowly working up to holding for 10 to 15 seconds.

If at first you are unable to grasp around your knee, try cradling your hands under your thigh.

If this is too difficult, place your foot on a small stool or pillow in front of you.

ADVANCED

1. Stand with your back resting against a wall.

2. Lift your leg and grasp just below the knee.

3. Slowly pull your knee upward toward your body. Hold for a count of 10 and then bring your leg back down.

4. Rest and repeat with your other leg.

As you progress, try holding your leg for up to 20 to 30 seconds.

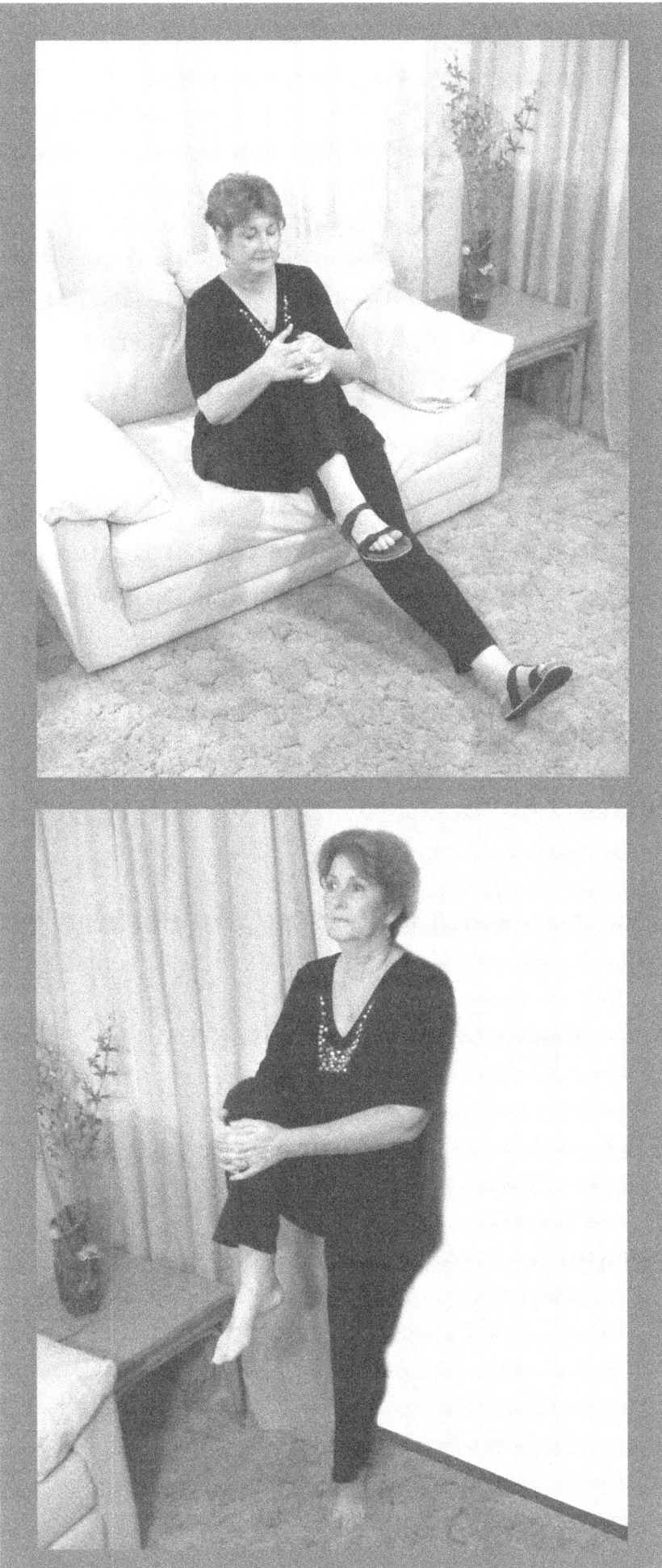

FACIAL CONTORTIONS

Laugh if you want, but we actually begin to lose muscle strength in our faces as well. So please, laugh if you want, whenever you want! Laughing is not only beneficial to your health; from lowering your blood pressure to giving your diaphragm muscles a good workout, to relieving stress. Many scientific studies not only back this up, but also point out that facial skin tone is improved with the stretching of the muscles.

1. Start by breaking into a big grin with your eyes wide open. Open your mouth and roll your eyes around. Pull your lips back and bare your teeth, feeling free to growl. Now close your mouth and relax.

2. Look forward, open your mouth wide and stick out your tongue, slowly moving it in and out and from side to side. Try sweeping the roof, floor, and sides of your mouth with it.

3. Stretch your face in a combination of smiles, grimaces and frowns. Roll your eyes and make sure you get your eyebrows into the act as well.

Be cautious for dizziness and be careful not to overstrain your eye muscles.

Have a ball! No one is looking, and if they are, have them join in the fun.

Have you had any water recently? If not, please have some.

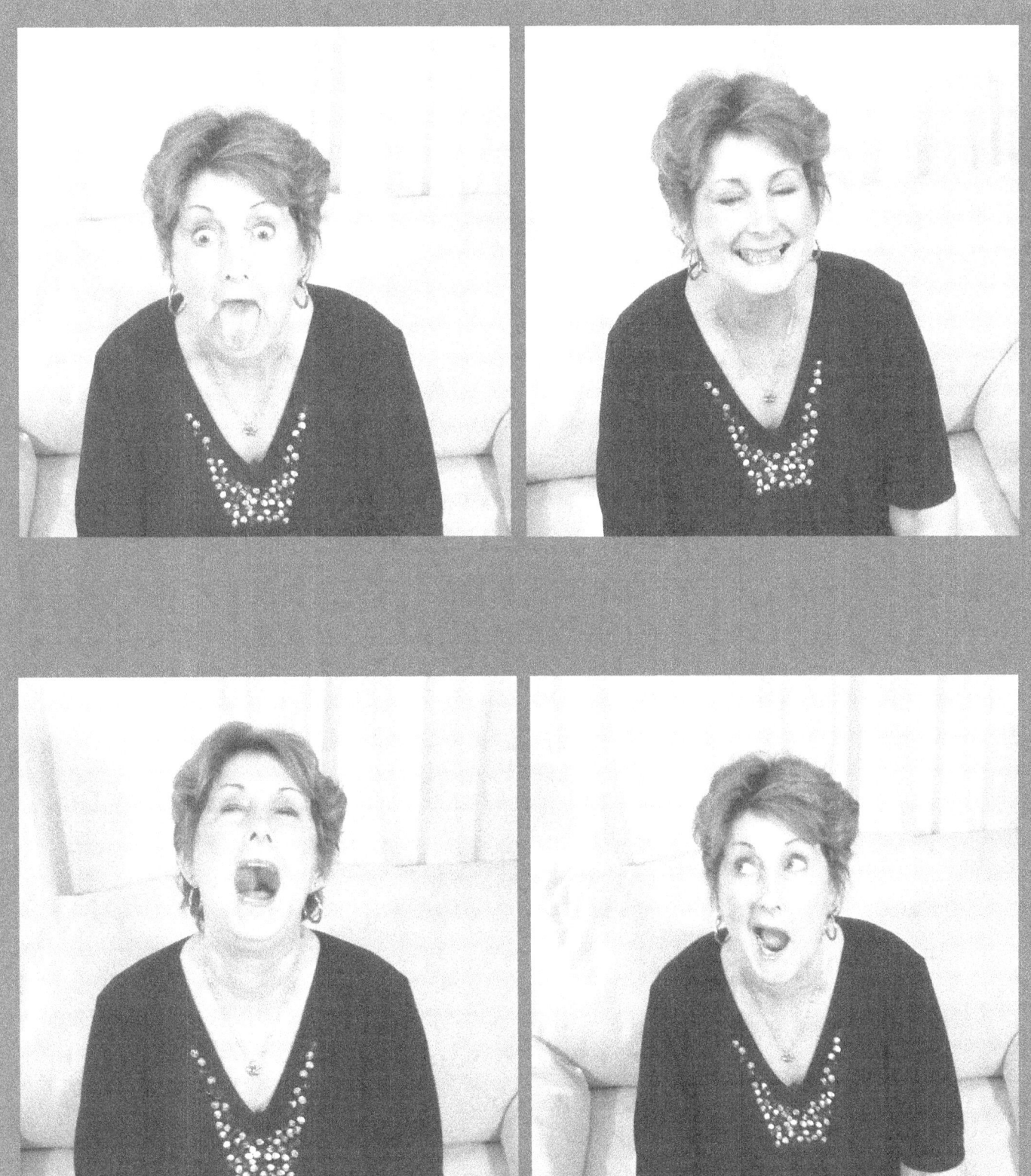

These exercises are beneficial to both men, women, and children, too. And you are encouraged to perform at whatever level is comfortable for you.

I want you to become stronger and more fit, but this comes with time and overdoing it at first will only cause you discomfort, disappointment, and ultimately disillusionment and failure.

So please be patient and it really won't be that long before you start to see the benefits.

Now let's get down to some
STRENGTH BUILDING

LEG LIFTS

1. Sit at the front of your seat with your arms grasping the edge, and your legs out in front with your knees straight.

2. Lift one leg up just a few inches off the ground and hold that position for a count of three. Return and lift the other.

Do three repetitions to start and then increase height and the time held.

Once you have built up strength, move back in your seat, and try doing it without holding on with your hands. This will benefit your stomach muscles and balance.

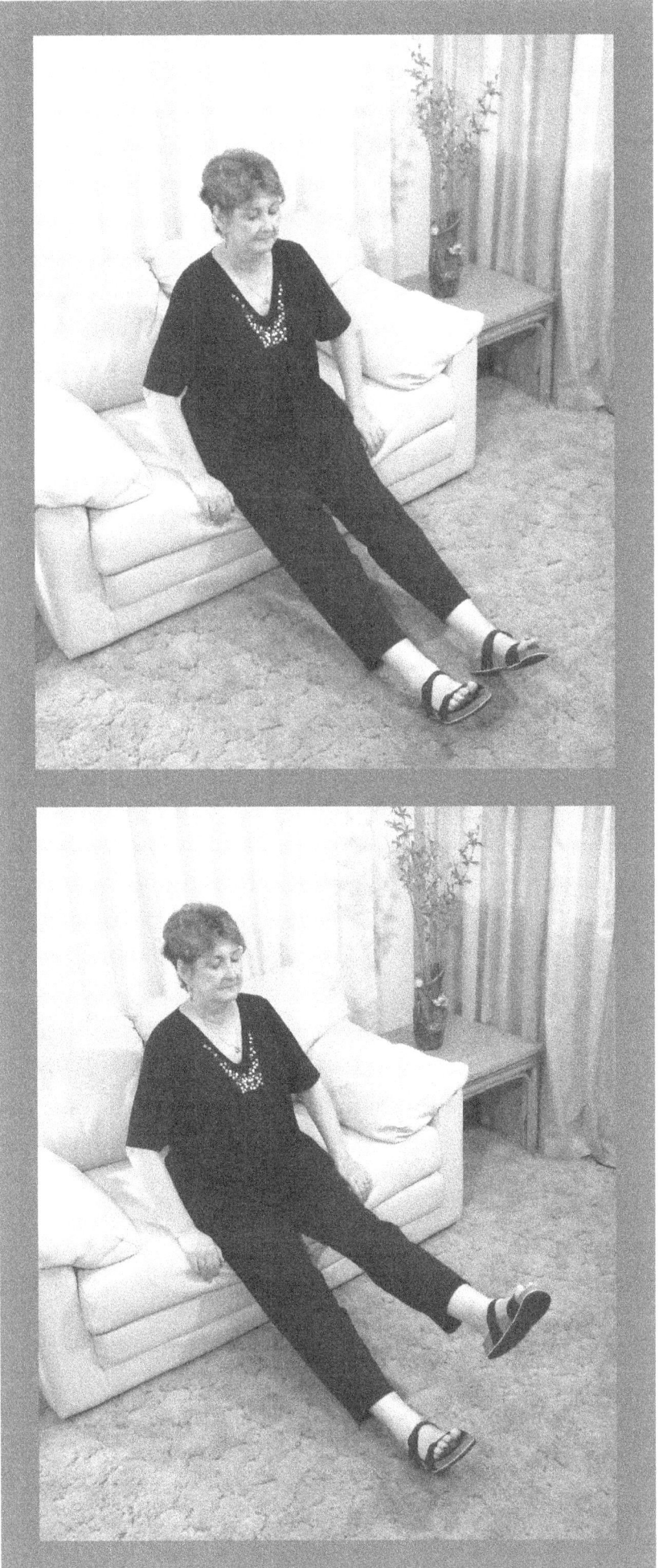

TOE LIFTS

1. Stand in front of your couch, with your feet a few inches apart.

2. Spread your arms out to the side and lift up on both feet so only your toes are on the floor. Hold for a three count and then return slowly to starting position.

Repeat this three times. As you progress, hold for 10 to 15 seconds.

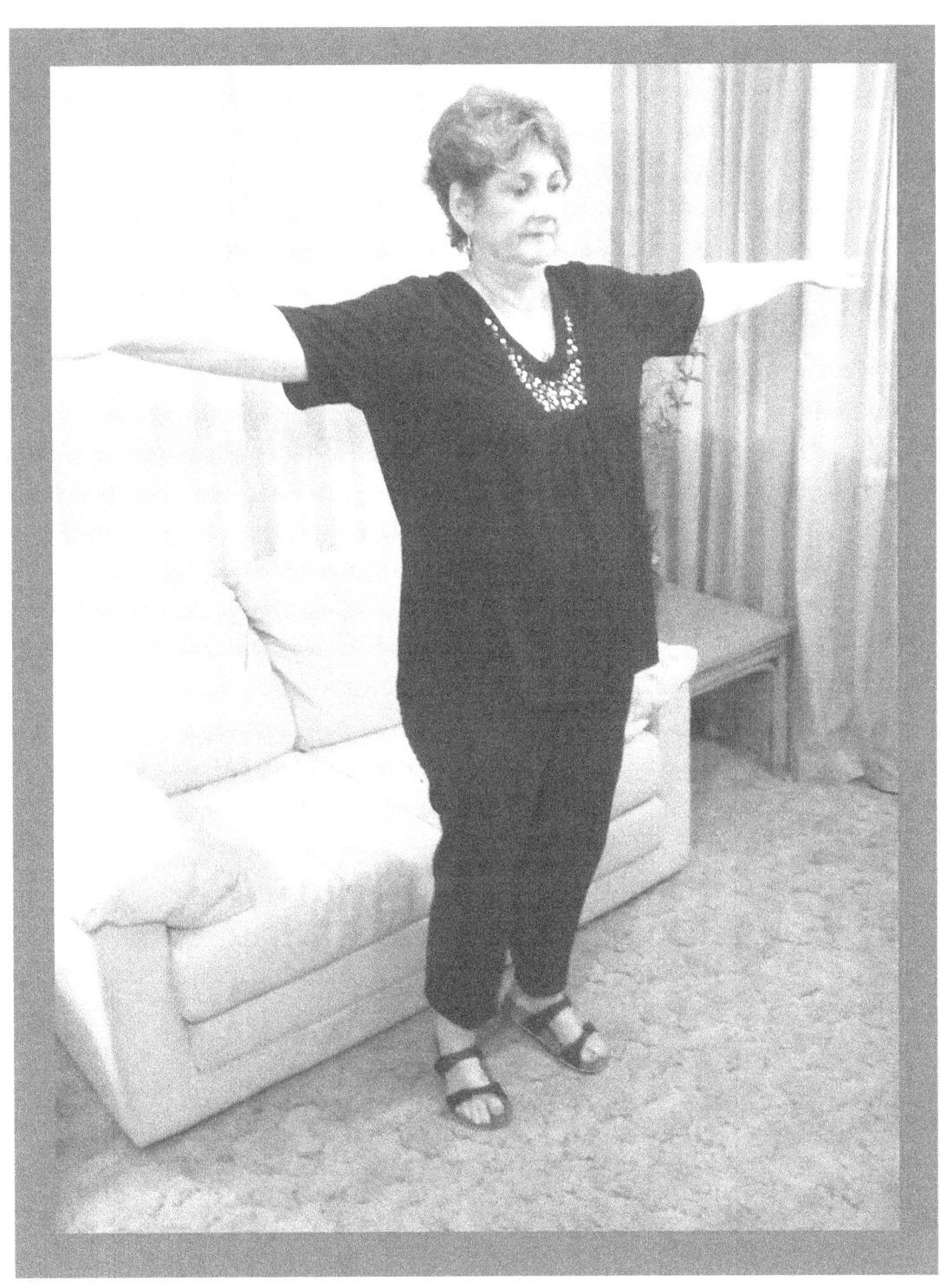

GRIP STRENGTHENING

1. Hold your hands in front of you with palms up and fingers wide open.

2. Very slowly close your fingers, resisting the motion, until you make a fist.

3. Unfold your hands using the same resistance.

Do three repetitions on each hand to start with, and increase to 10 or more.

Eventually you can move on to squeezing a small rubber ball, a rolled up towel, or even a newspaper.

1. Put it in your hand and squeeze it, holding the squeeze for a count of three, releasing and repeating five times.

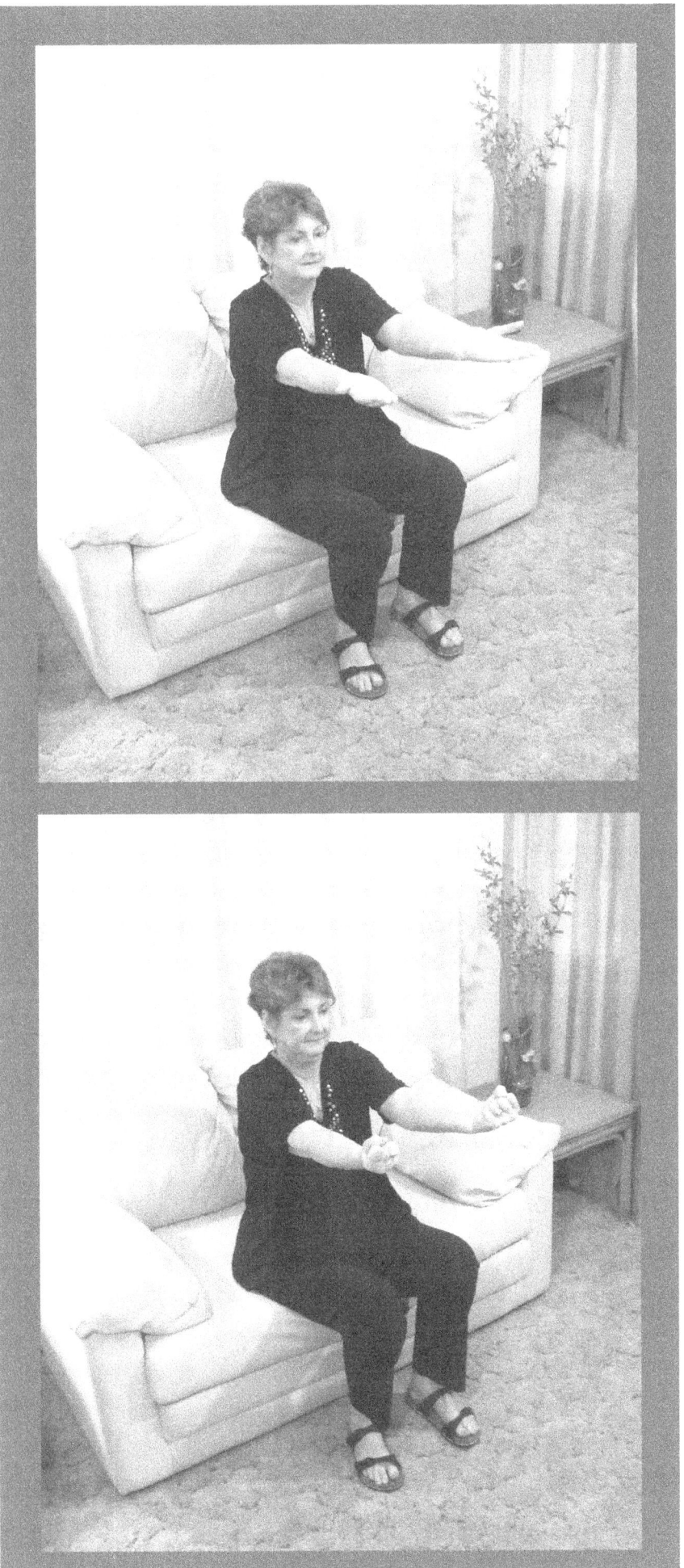

BICEPS CURLS

1. Sit on the front of the couch with your knees bent and feet flat on the floor.

2. Stretch out your left arm, make a fist, and slowly bend at the elbow, bringing your fist up toward your shoulder as you resist the motion.

Start with three repetitions for each hand.

After doing this for a few weeks or so:

1. Place your right hand on the top of the fist.

2. Slowly, bend your elbow and bring your fist up toward your shoulder while applying only slight resistance with the right hand.

3. Push the left hand back with the right hand, applying resistance with the left. Repeat with other hand.

Start with three repetitions for each hand. Increasing repetitions and amount of resistance as your strength grows.

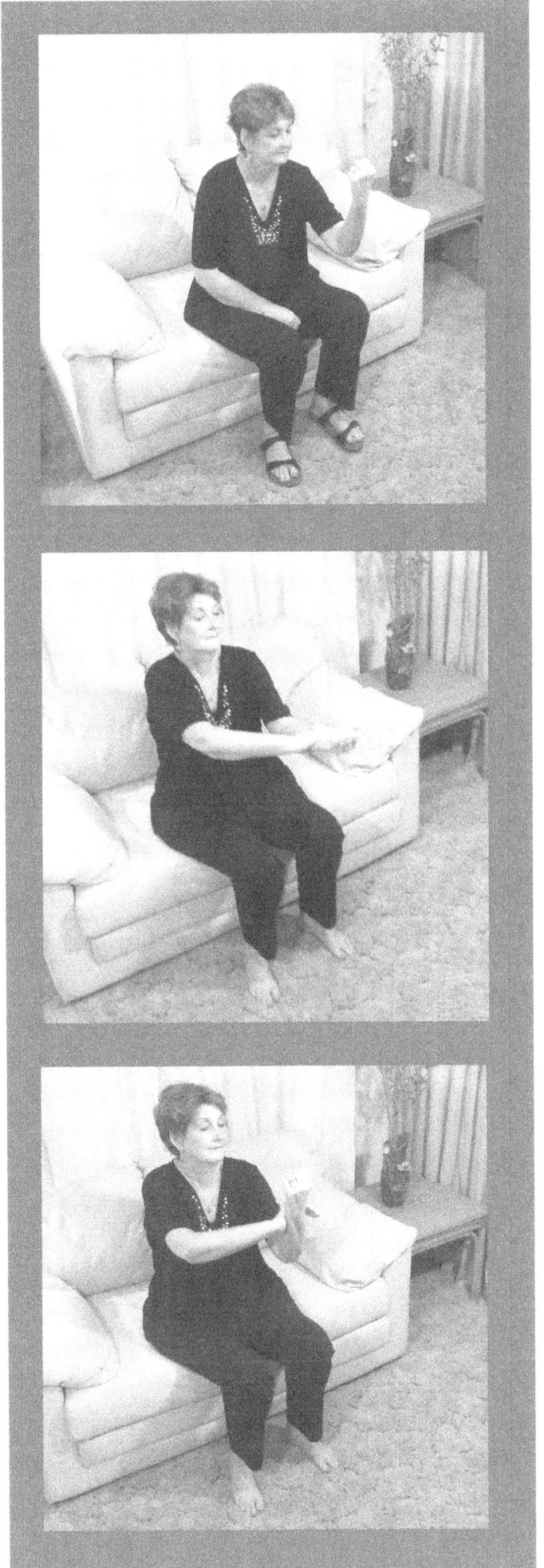

TRICEPS CURLS

1. Bring your left fist near your ear with your elbow pointing out in front of you and your fingers facing up.

2. Bring your right hand over and cover your fist with it.

3. Extend your fist upward while resisting with your right hand.

Do three repetitions and then switch arms.

Increase repetitions and resistance force as your strength develops.

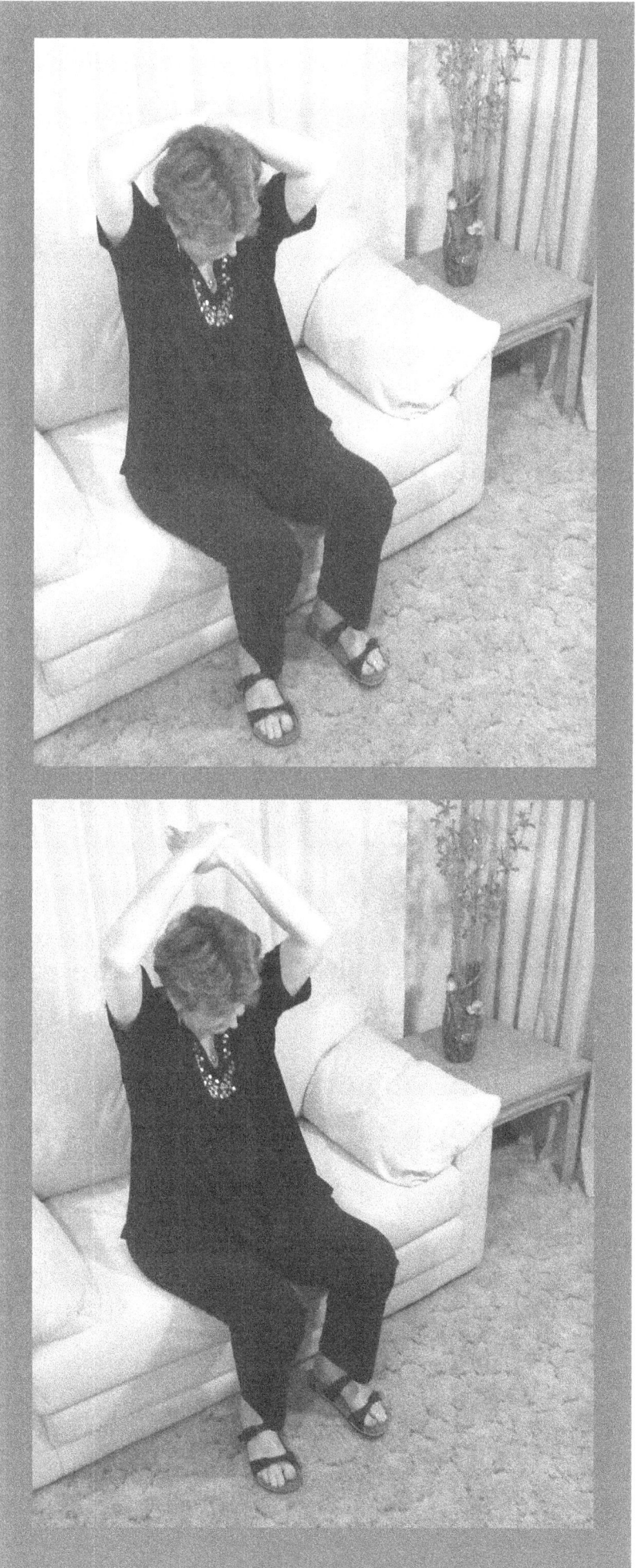

LOWER ARM ROTATIONS

1. Find an object with a short, round handle, or a rolled up magazine with a rubber band around the middle.

2. Extend your arms part way with the object in both hands like small handlebars.

3. Slowly rotate the object using your hands in an alternate spinning motion, as if you were winding it upward.

Do this for five seconds to start and increase time over a period of weeks.

ADVANCED

1. Tie a three-foot string to the middle of the rolled-up object and attach it to a small weight.

2. Sit or stand. Wind the object up until the weight is all the way to the top, and then slowly unwind until it reaches the bottom.

Repeat, adding repetitions and adjust time to suit your advancement.

You can increase the weight of the object, but the motion alone will be beneficial.

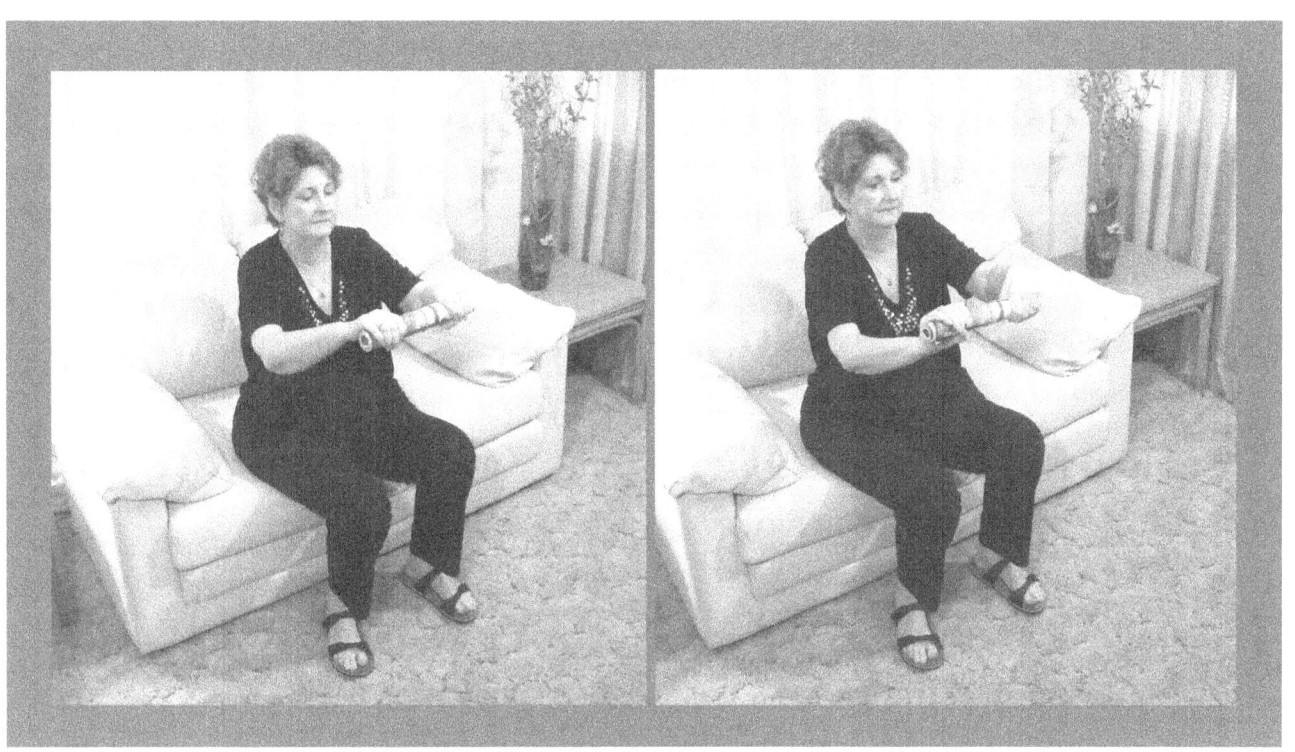

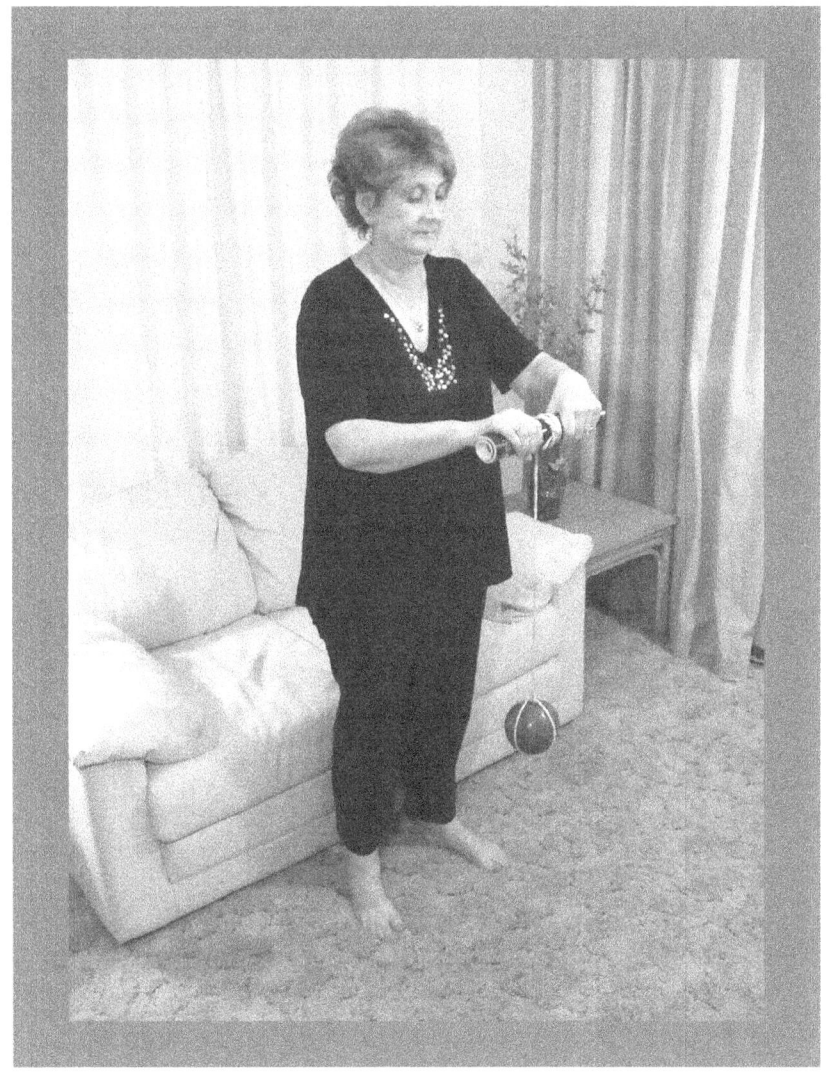

PADDLING

1. Stand with your legs shoulder width apart or sit at the edge of your couch and arms at your side.

2. Raise your arms out to the side as high is comfortable.

Do five repetitions to start and don't flap or flail!

As your stamina increases, increase reps and speed until you feel that you can last for 20 to 30 seconds.

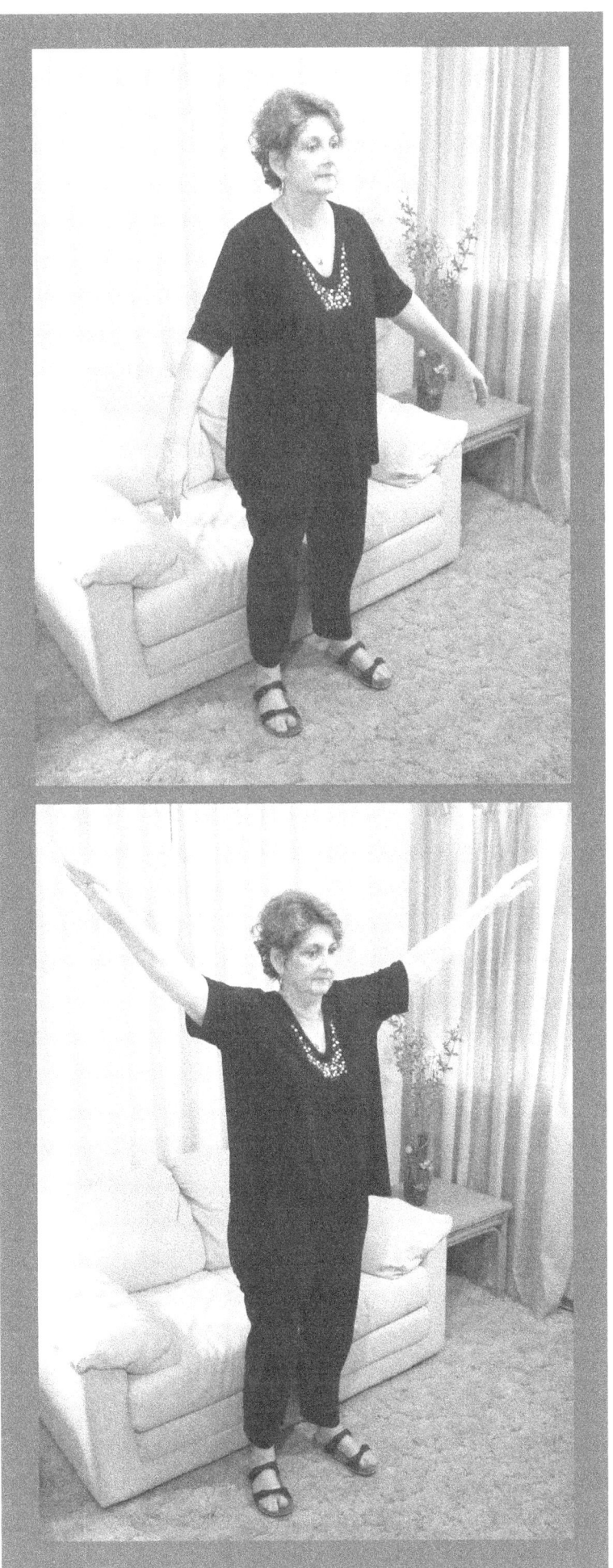

PUNCHING

1. Sit at the edge of the couch, or stand with knees slightly bent. Bring your upturned fists back, fingers up, until they are even with your torso and at the same height as your belly button.

2. Keep your shoulders back and slowly extend your right fist straight out at shoulder height, with fingers are facing down.

Your fist should have a slight downward angle and you should be able to look down your arm and over the top of your hand and not see your knuckles.

3. Retract your fist to the original position. At the same time extend the left one.

Rest and repeat three times for each hand.

Advance by increasing the speed of punches, and number of repetitions. As strength and endurance increases, try doing this exercise with resistance in slow motion and straining against yourself as you move.

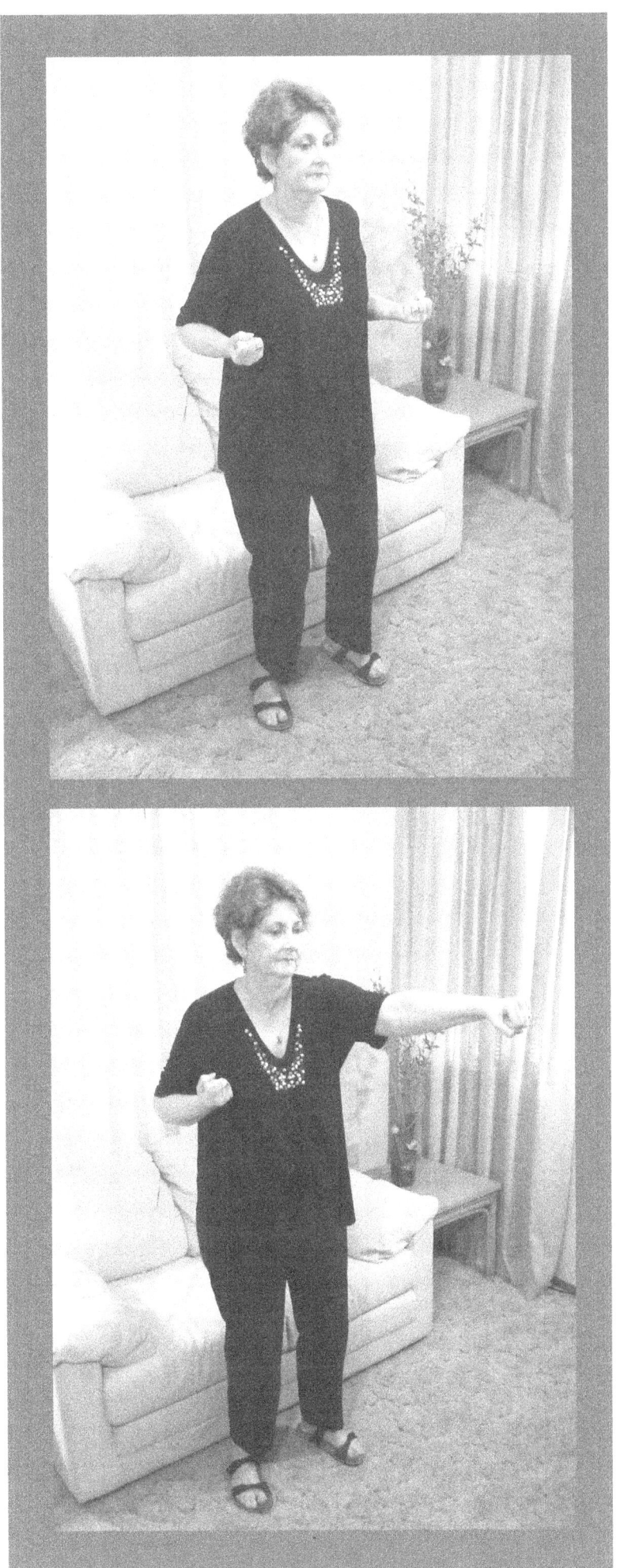

BENT LEG LIFTS

1. Sit or stand with your arms at your sides and your feet flat on the floor.

2. Slowly lift and lower your right knee.

3. Repeat with left knee.

Begin with three sets of three lifts each and increase over time.

For an advanced posture lift your leg to a comfortable height, extend it and hold.

LEG LIFTS, SINGLE

1. Sit with both hands grasping the arms or front of your seat, with feet flat on the floor.

2. Slowly extend the left leg until it is in the air.

3. Hold for a three count. Alternate legs.

Start with three repetitions for each leg.

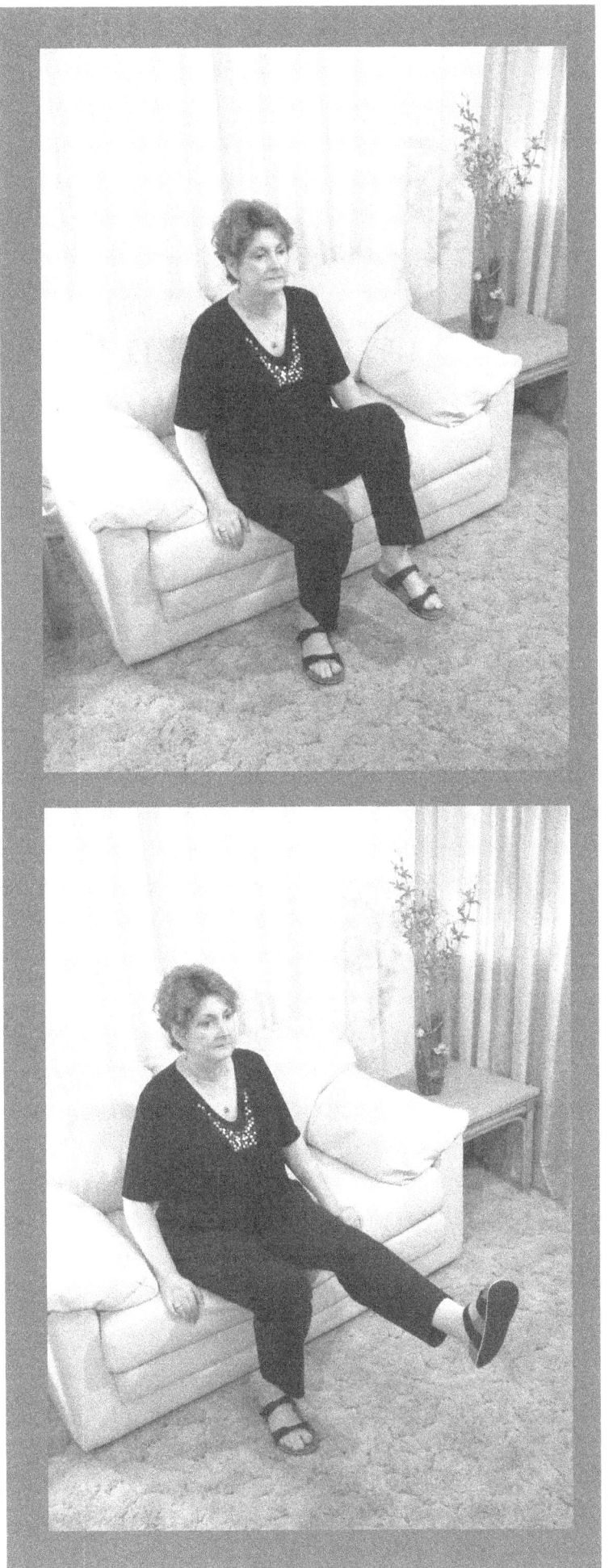

ADVANCED LEG LIFTS/ABDOMINAL

1. Sit slightly forward on your couch with your legs straight out and your heels on floor.

2. Grasp the arms of your couch or chair or place hands at the back of the seat and slowly raise both legs off the floor. (This requires a little bit of leaning back.)

3. Hold for a count of three and then return feet to floor.

As you get stronger, increase the height of your legs and duration of the exercise.

FOR ADDED STRENGTH

After you are comfortable with the advanced lifts try this:

1. Extend your legs, spread your feet apart and hold.

2. Start by counting to three and keep adding time as you get better.

REMEMBER TO DO ONLY WHAT YOU CAN AT ANY GIVEN TIME AND DON'T OVER DO IT!

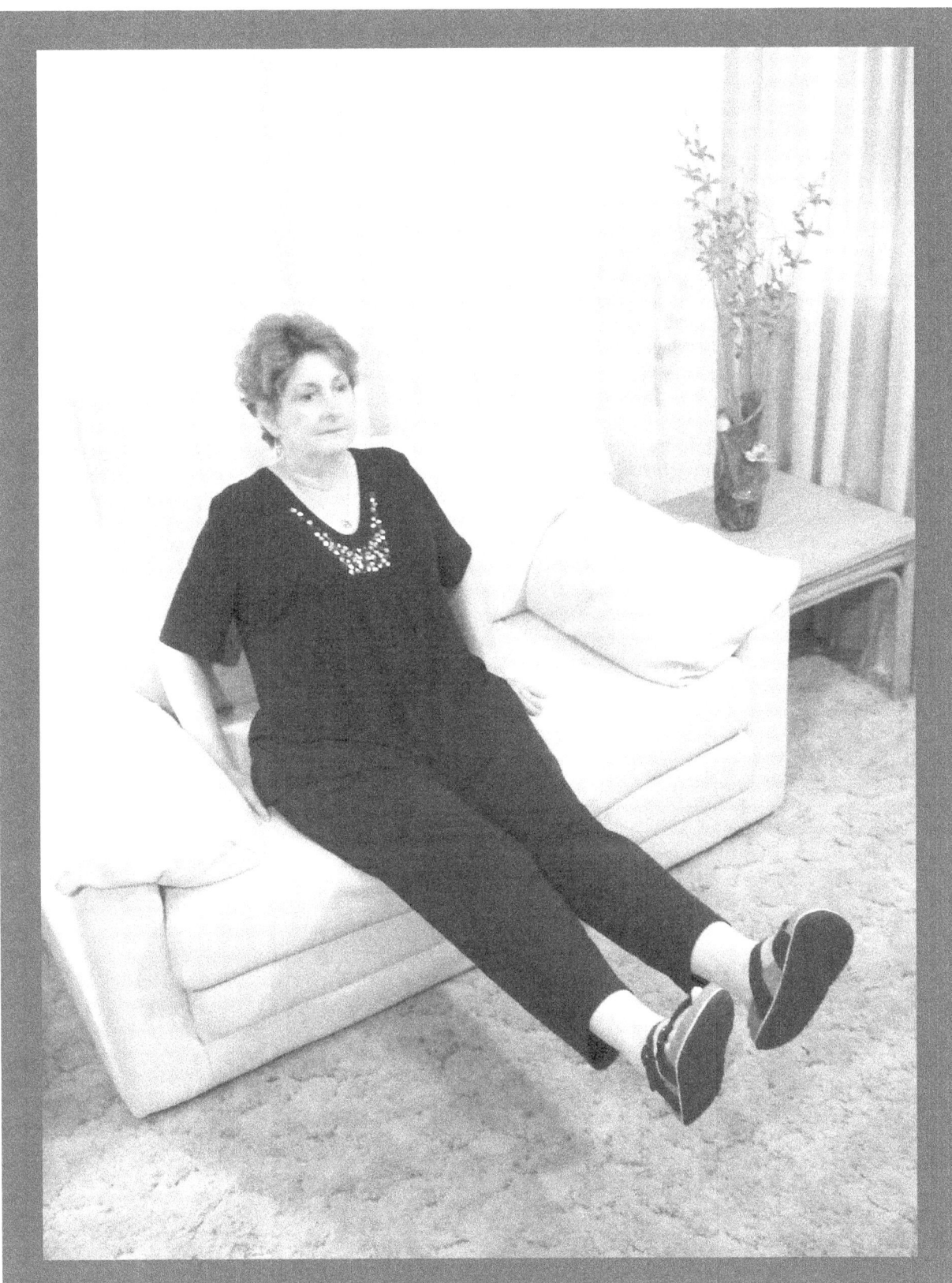

SIT BACKS

1. Sit at the front of the couch with your arms crossed loosely over your chest. Stretch your legs out comfortably in front of you, with feet flat on the floor.

2. Slowly lean back until you are touching the couch, inhaling as you go.

3. Keep your feet flat on the floor and sit forward with your arms still crossed, exhaling.

Repeat this three times and keep increasing repetitions as time goes by.

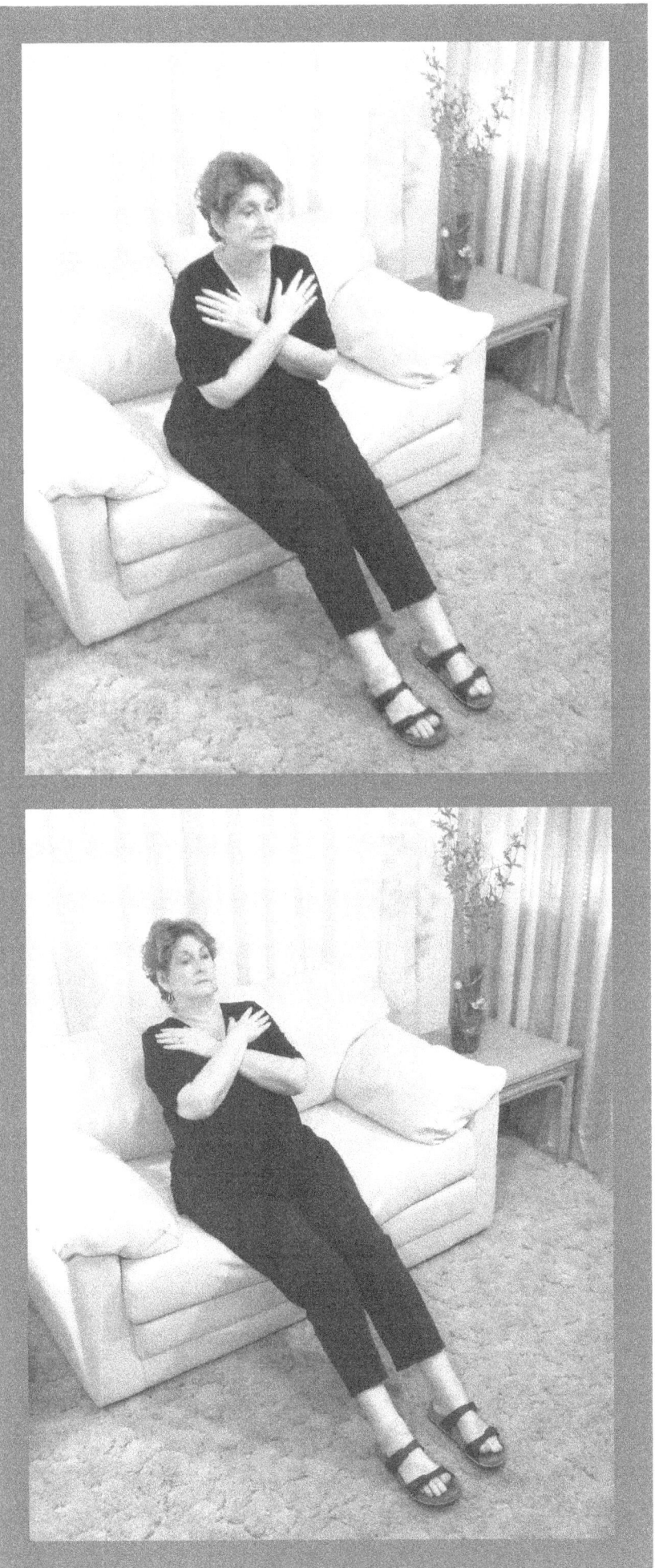

SHOULDER AND CHEST STRENGTHENING

1. Place heels of palms together in front of your chest with fingers on the other wrist.

2. Slowly push the left arm to the right, at the same time resisting with the right hand.

3. Once your left hand is in front of your right shoulder, push to the left with your right hand, resisting with the left.

4. Go to the other side using the same method.

Repeat this three times, increasing repetitions, distance, and resistance.

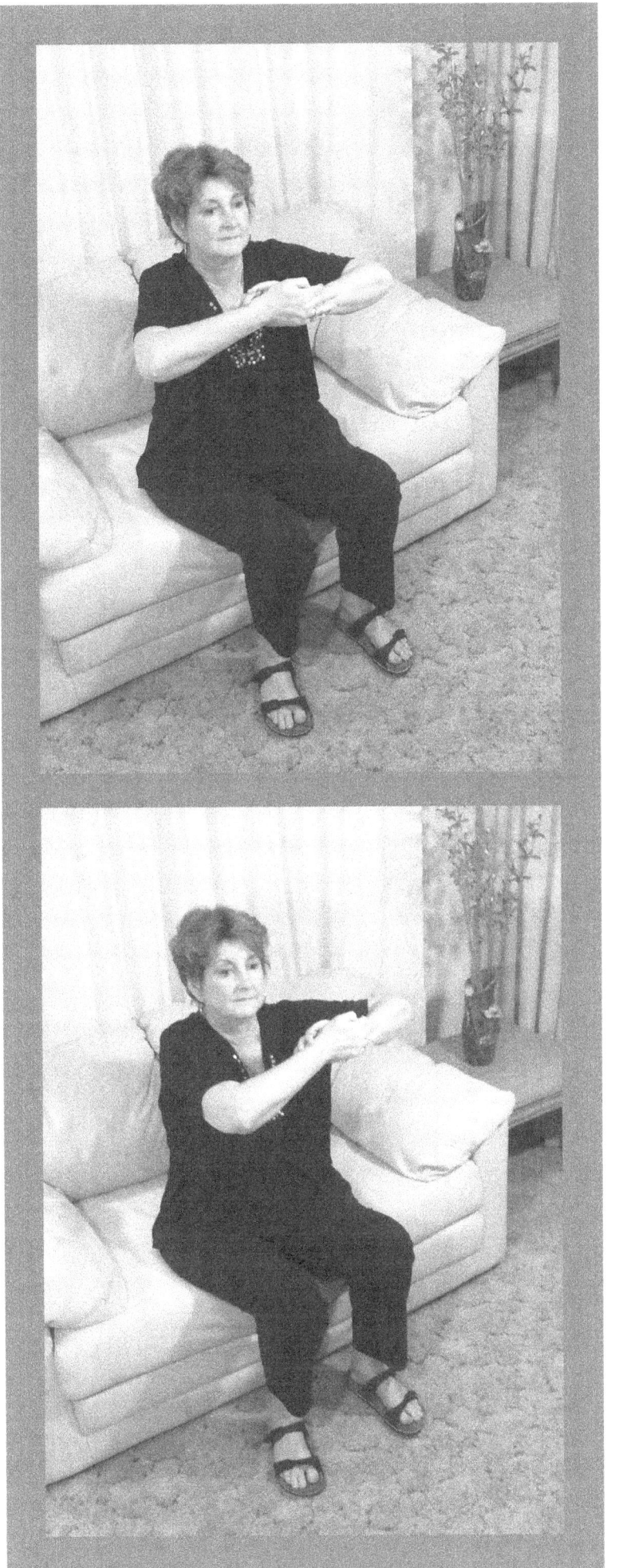

WALL PUSH

1. Stand arm's length from the wall.

2. Tilt forward keeping your back straight and palms against the wall slightly wider than shoulder width.

3. Slowly compress toward the wall, inhaling. Push away slowly as you exhale until you are back in starting position.

Do three pushes and then rest.

Add one more set of three if you feel up to it.

Increase number of repetitions and move feet away from the wall as strength and stamina allow.

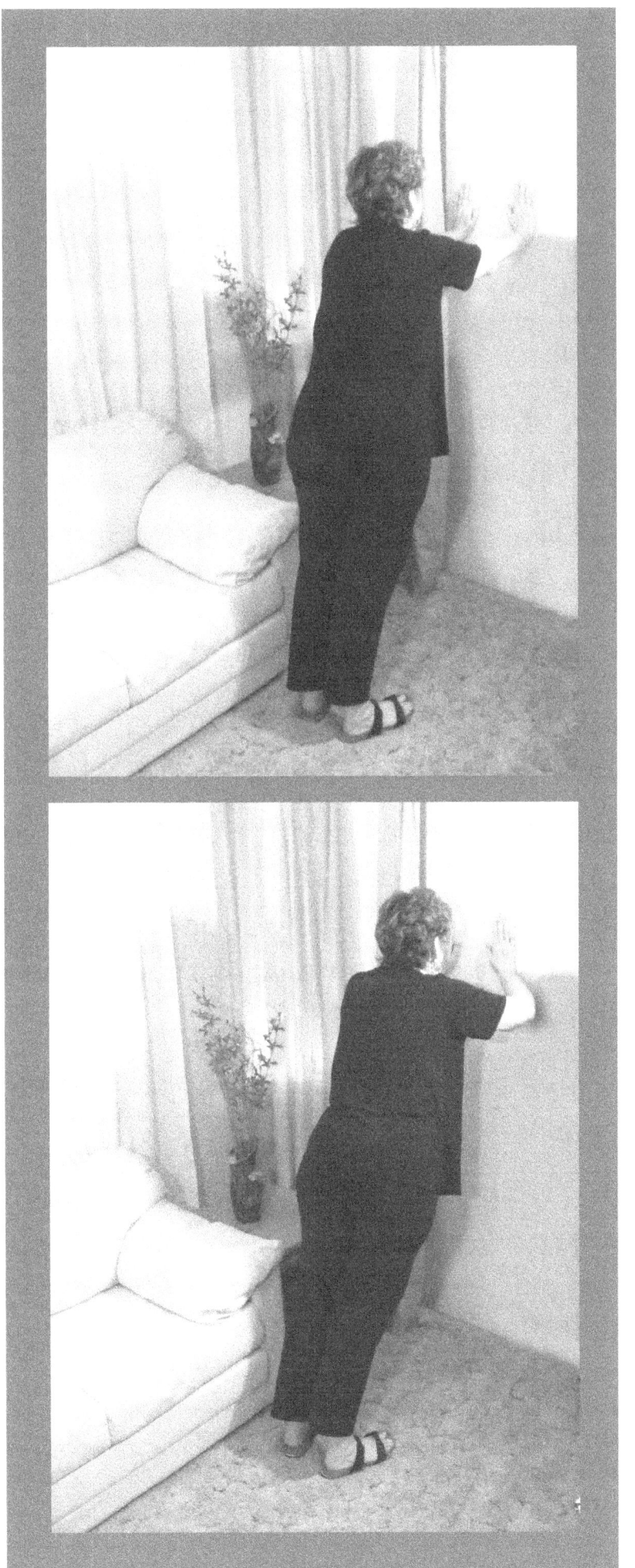

SQUATS

1. Stand in front of the couch with your feet shoulder width apart and your heels touching the couch.

2. Extend your arms out straight and bend at the knees slightly. Go down only as comfort and balance will allow.

3. Immediately return to upright position.

Repeat three times. (The couch behind you is your safety net should you have any balance issues.)

As you progress, try to remain in the squat for a count of three. You may continue to increase time and depth of squats as you improve. The goal is to eventually squat down almost to sitting on the couch and return to standing without having to touch the couch with your arms.

This exercise puts strain on your thighs and buttocks as well as your midsection.

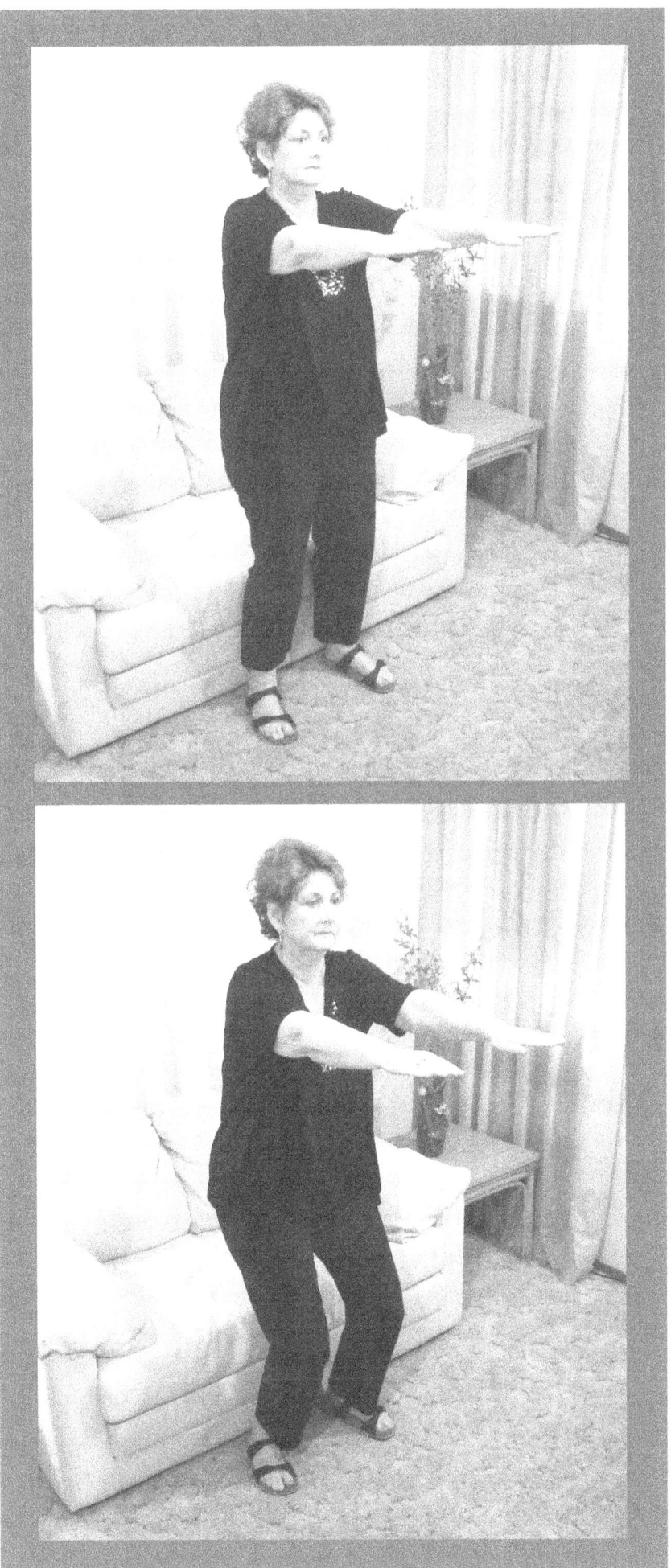

AEROBIC FINISH

Feeling like you did something? Good!

1. Walk in place right in front of your couch or chair for at least three to five minutes.

2. Make sure to bend your arms and swing them as if you were climbing a hill.

It would be great if someday you could walk for 20 to 30 minutes, but that goal is entirely up to you and your stamina.

Here is an alternative, if you don't feel up to walking.

SWAY

Turn off your TV and turn on the radio, or put on some of your favorite music. There is a great benefit to having your whole body moving and a little dancing can help you achieve that.

1. Start swaying gently to the beat, barely swaying at first.

2. Keep your eyes open to avoid any balance problems and just let the music move you.

This is a great way to cool down after you complete your workout.

Remember to slow down at the end of your swaying to allow your heart, breathing and blood flow to return to normal.

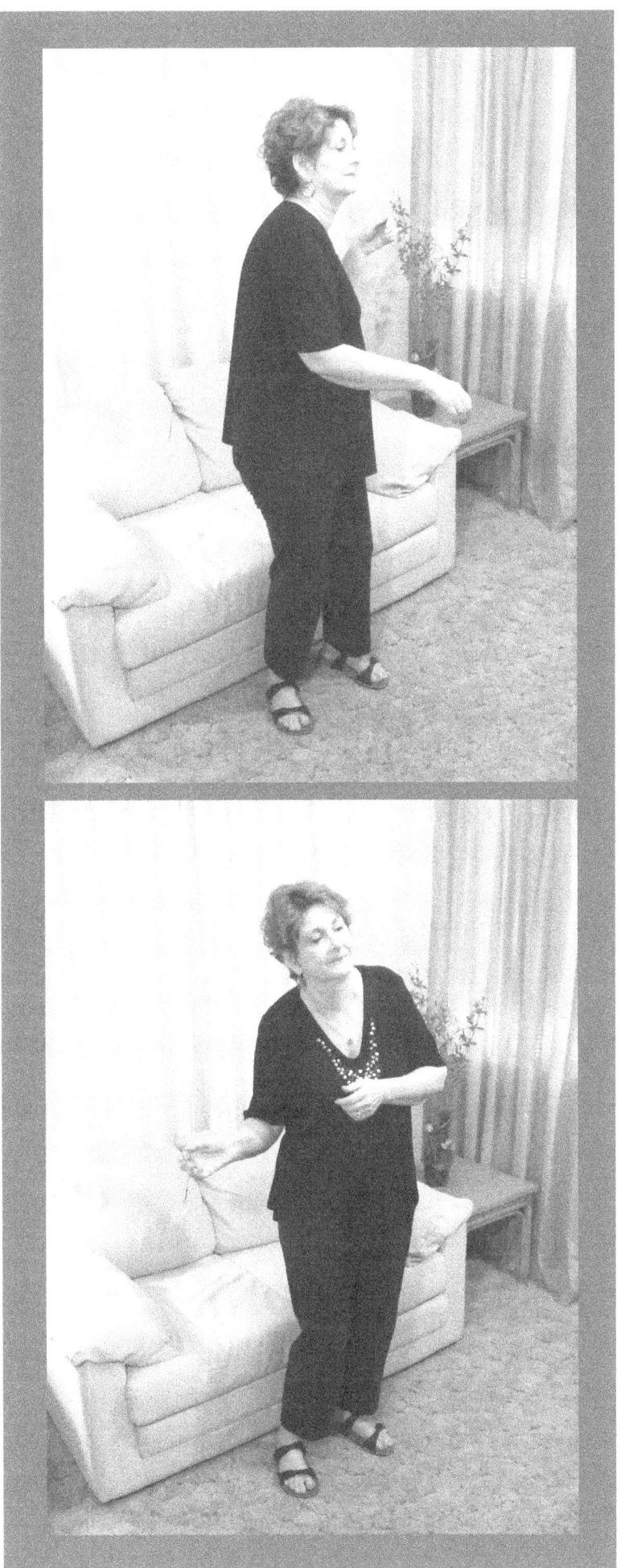

ADVANCED EXERCISES

These exercises are for those who have advanced, and are comfortable lying flat on the floor or stepping away from the couch.

You must always be honest with yourself and never go beyond what you are capable of doing.

If you strain something it will not only cause a break in your regimen but even worse, a break in your spirit, and could possibly keep you from continuing, so please be patient.

TOE TOUCHES

1. Stand with legs spread a little more than shoulder width apart and your arms outstretched to the side.

2. Reach across with your right hand and touch as far down your left leg as you can. The goal is to reach your ankle or your foot.

3. Return to standing and then repeat with left hand.

Start with counting to five and increase your depth and duration as you progress.

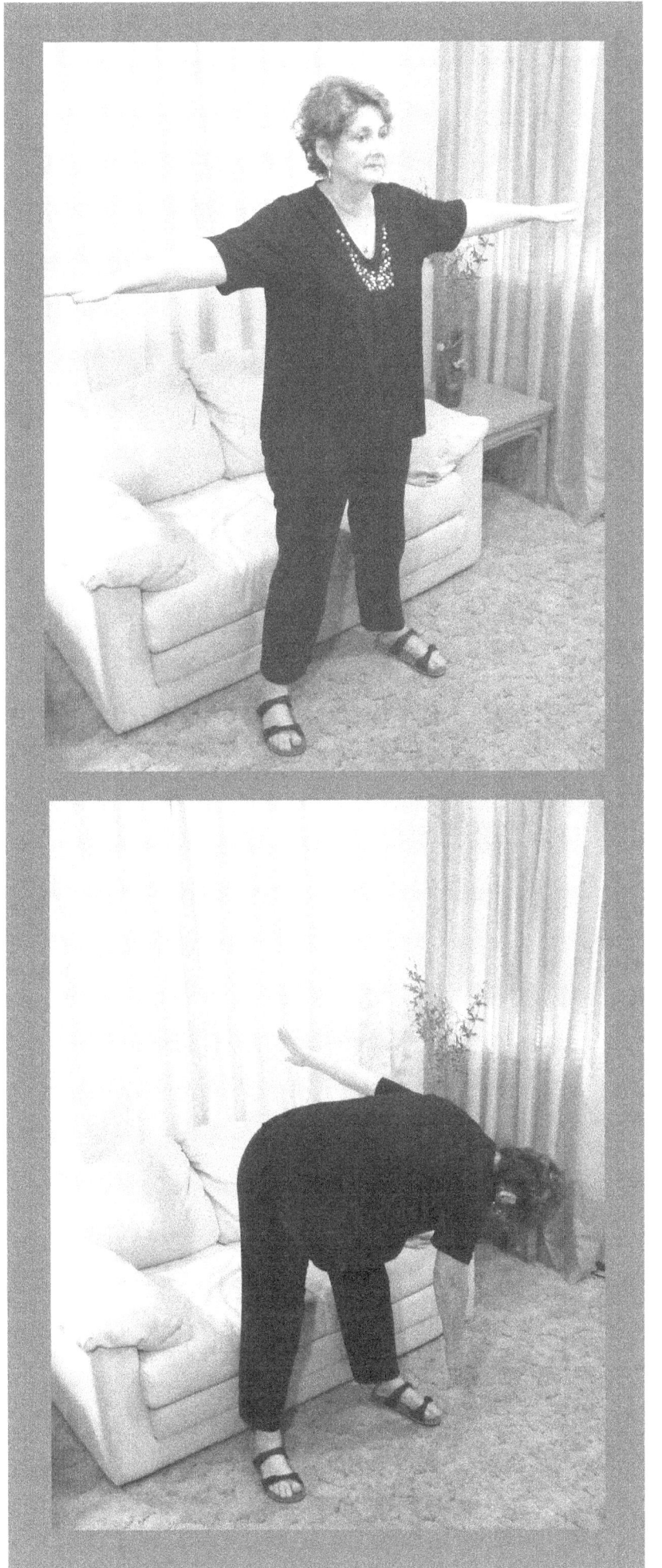

"PUSH PUPS"

1. Lie face down on the floor with your palms down just outside your shoulders.

2. Slowly lift your torso just a few inches off the floor keeping your back straight and using your knees as the base.

3. Return to prone position.

Try to start with three and increase repetitions and height as you gain strength.

The goal is a full arm extension.

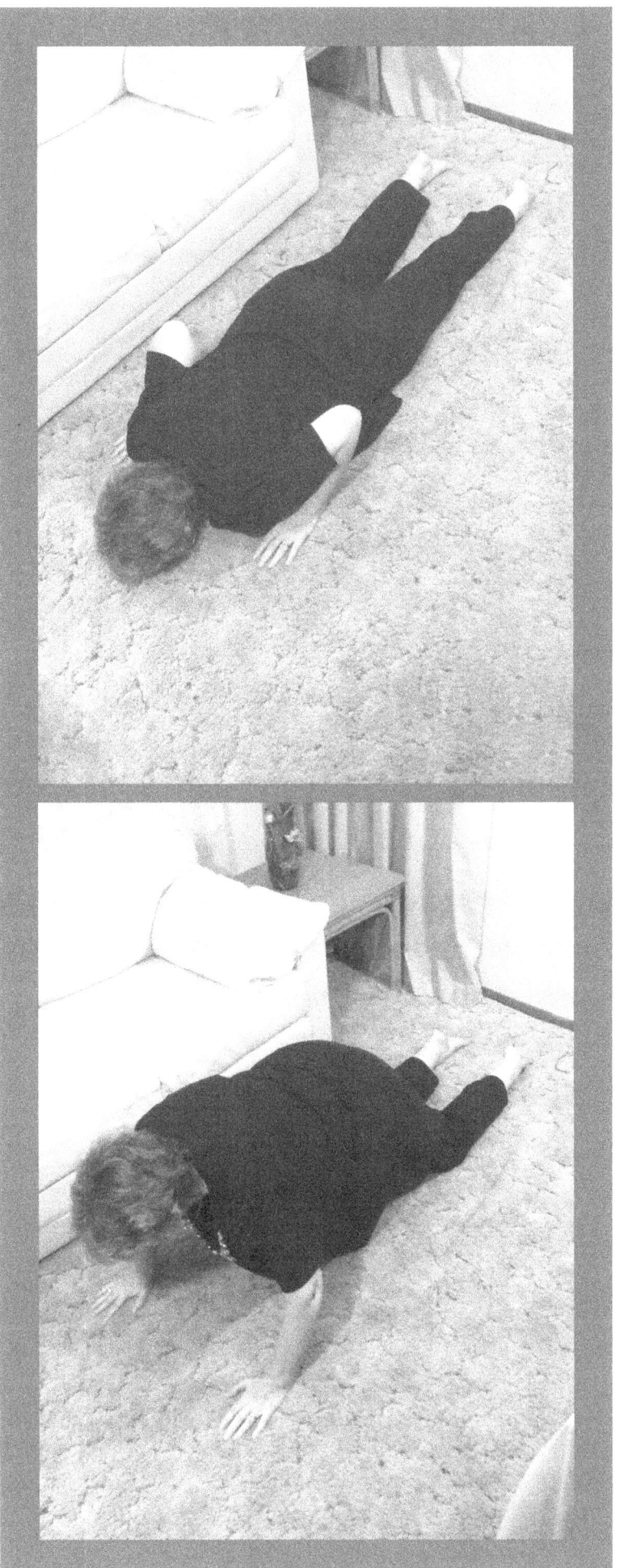

LEG LIFTS

1. Lie on your back with your hands palms down at your sides and your legs together.

2. Lift your legs as high as you can, eventually reaching a 45-degree angle.

3. Return them to the floor.

Start with a count of three.

Once you improve, try it with your hands clasped behind your head.

For extra strength, spread your legs as you lower them, leaving them about four to six inches off the floor. Hold that for a couple of seconds or as long as possible.

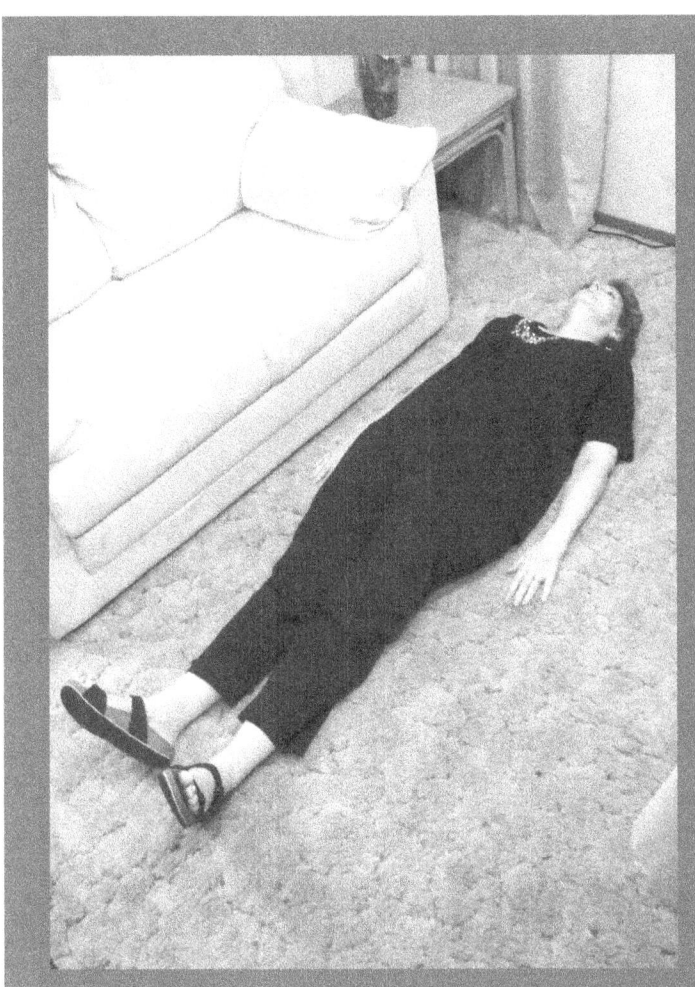
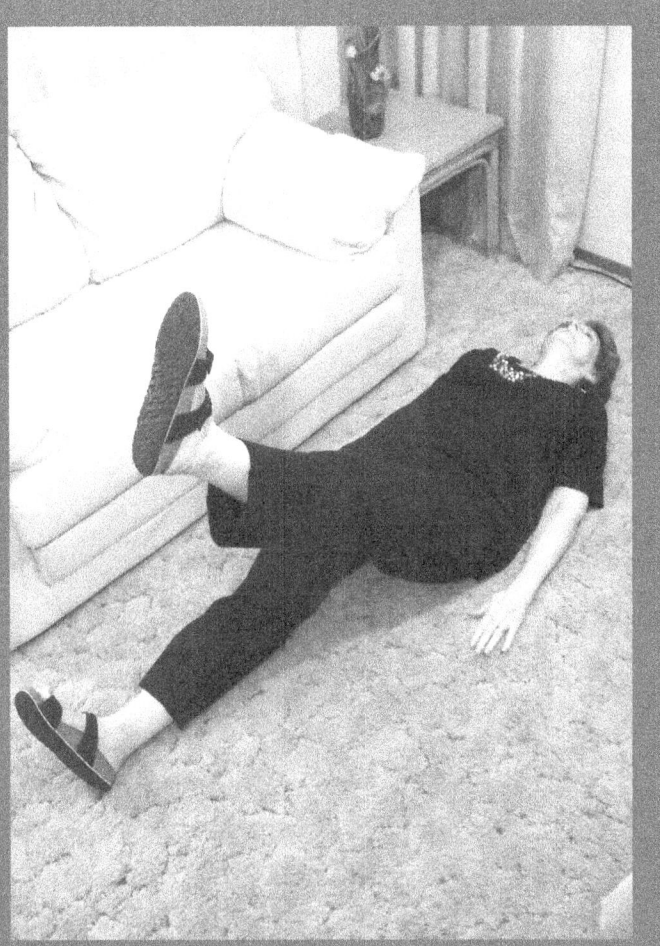
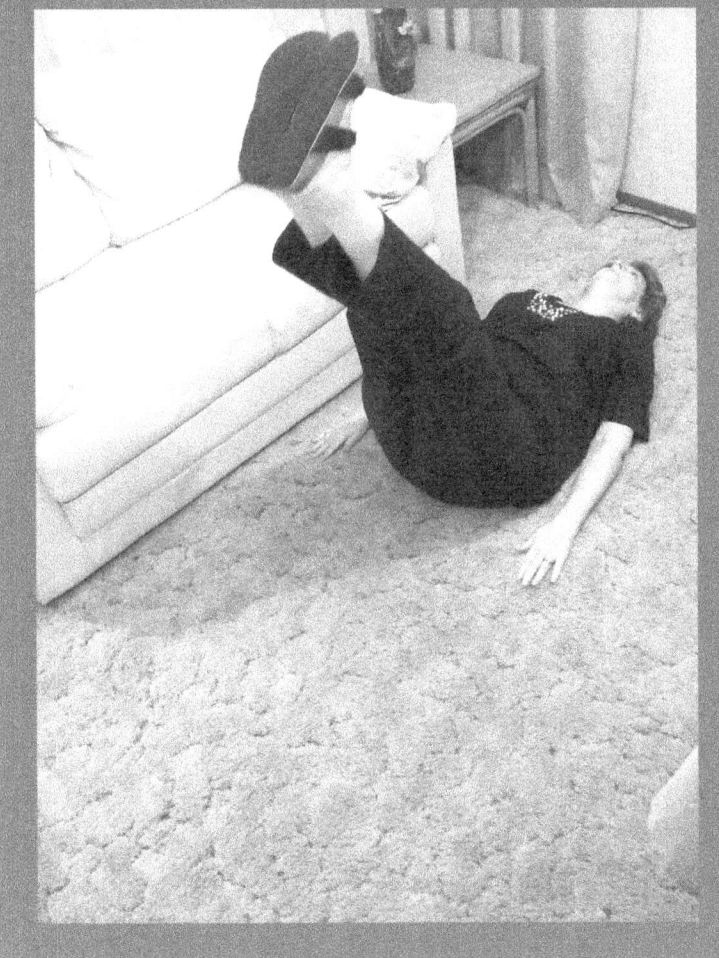

SIT UPS

1. Sit on the floor with your knees bent and your toes under the couch. Place a small pillow or folded blanket under your buttocks.

2. Lay back on the floor with your arms crossed on your chest.

3. Lift up to a sitting position and then lower back down.

Start with just one, two, or three and increase a few at a time only when you have mastered them.

Once you are able to do 20 sit ups, try turning to one side and then the other with each sit up. This will help to firm up your sides as well as your abdomen.

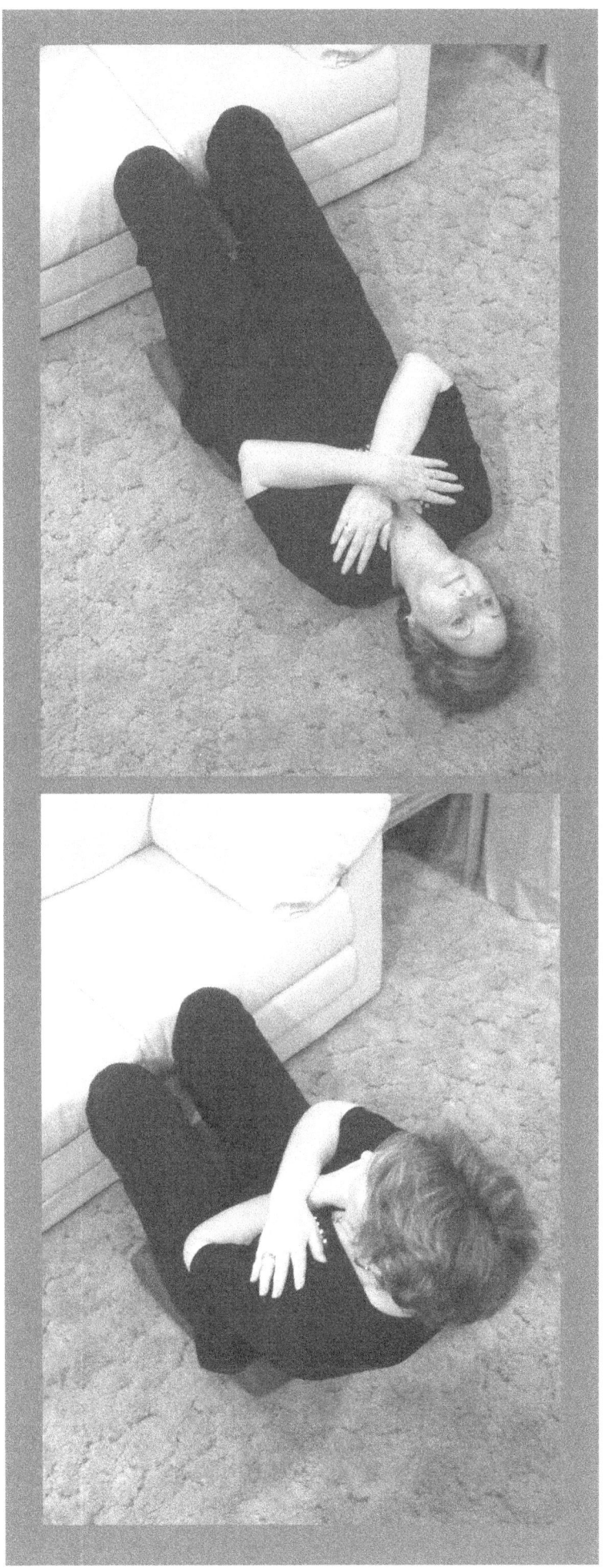

REAR AND THIGH

1. Get down on your hands and knees with your hands just a little wider than shoulder width.

2. Draw your left knee up toward your chest.

3. Slowly straighten your leg out behind you.

4. Once extended, bring it slowly back and rest it on the floor.

Repeat three times and then do the same with your right leg.

After you get stronger, you can increase the number of repetitions and keep your knee off the floor.

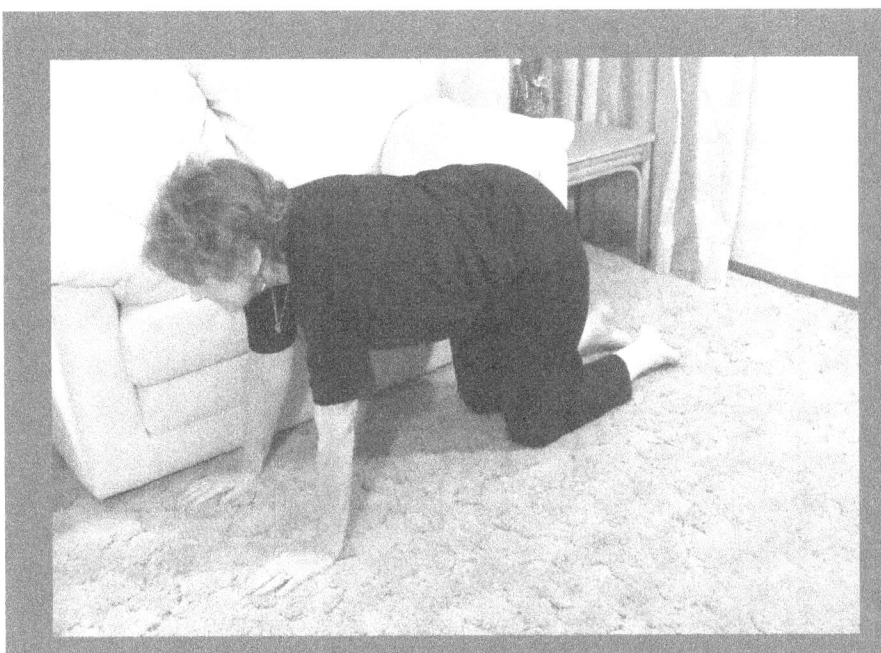

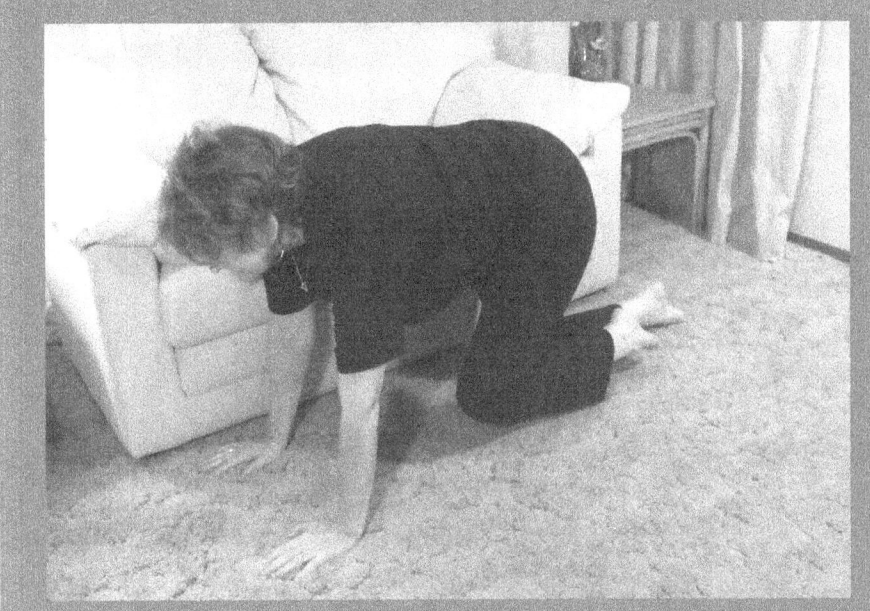

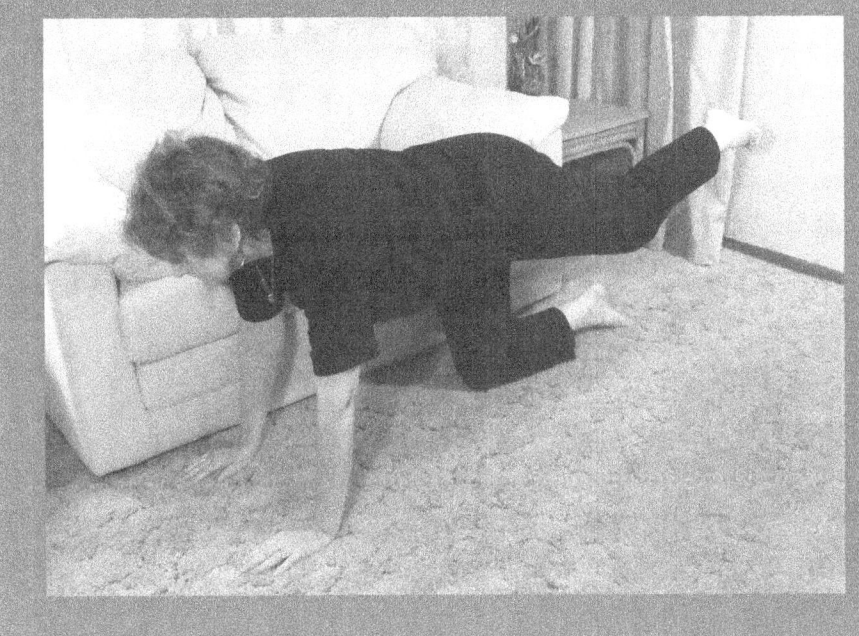

HIGH-STEP WALKING

1. Walk briskly in place, lifting your knees as high as you can and pump your arms at the same time.

Do this for at least two to three minutes and increase time when ready.

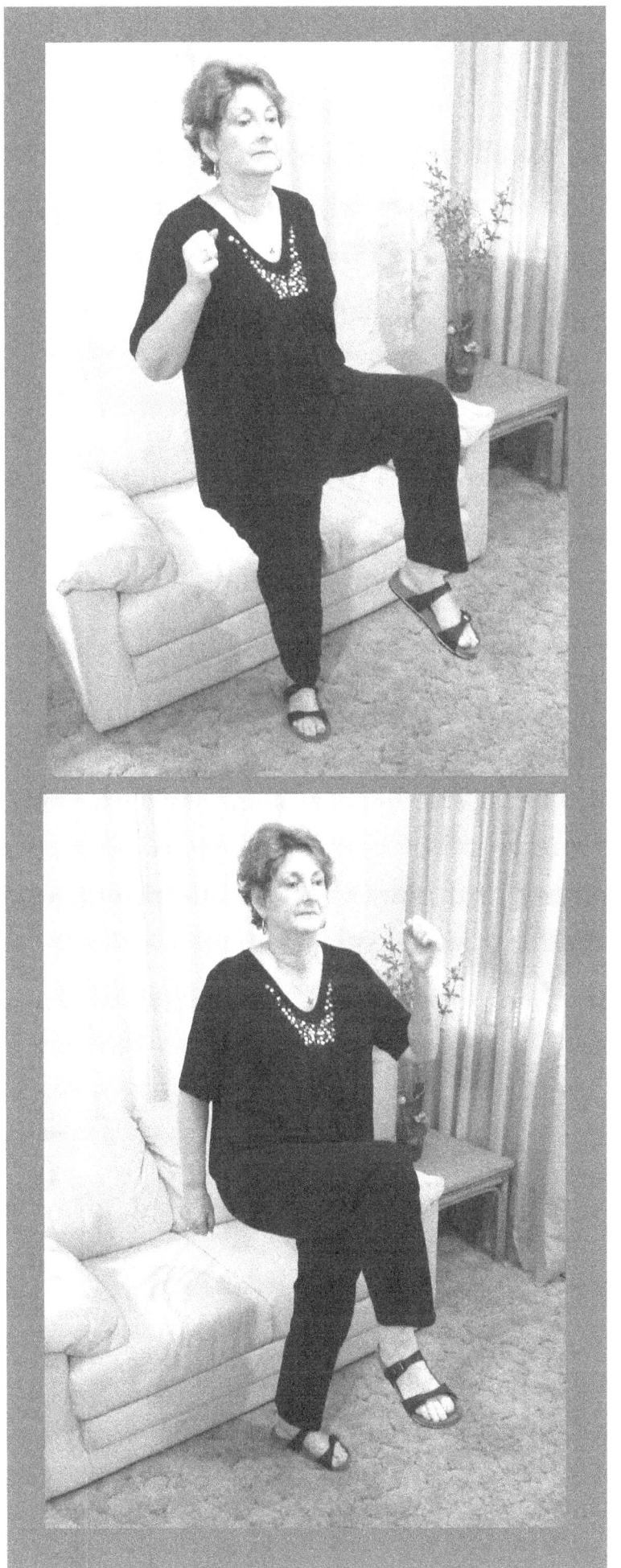

STAIRS

Do you live in a dwelling with a safe, well-lit stairway?

If so, and if you feel comfortable with it; try slowly walking up and down your stairs.

1. Make sure to always have one hand on the railing while going up and down.

2. Start with three to five minutes and work your way up as you feel your endurance and strength increasing.

A 20- to 30-minute workout would be tremendous, but don't rush into it. Remember this an advanced exercise.

One of the great benefits to stair walking is that you lift 70% of your body weight with each step and without any jarring impact on your joints.

A WORD OF CAUTION: This exercise has an element of danger and if at any time you feel light headed or dizzy, immediately sit down on the stairs and lean slightly back keeping one hand on the railing. Breathe normally.

Set a timer out of your sight and try passing the time by listening to your favorite music.

COOL DOWN

Always end your workout by walking in place or swaying for a few minutes.

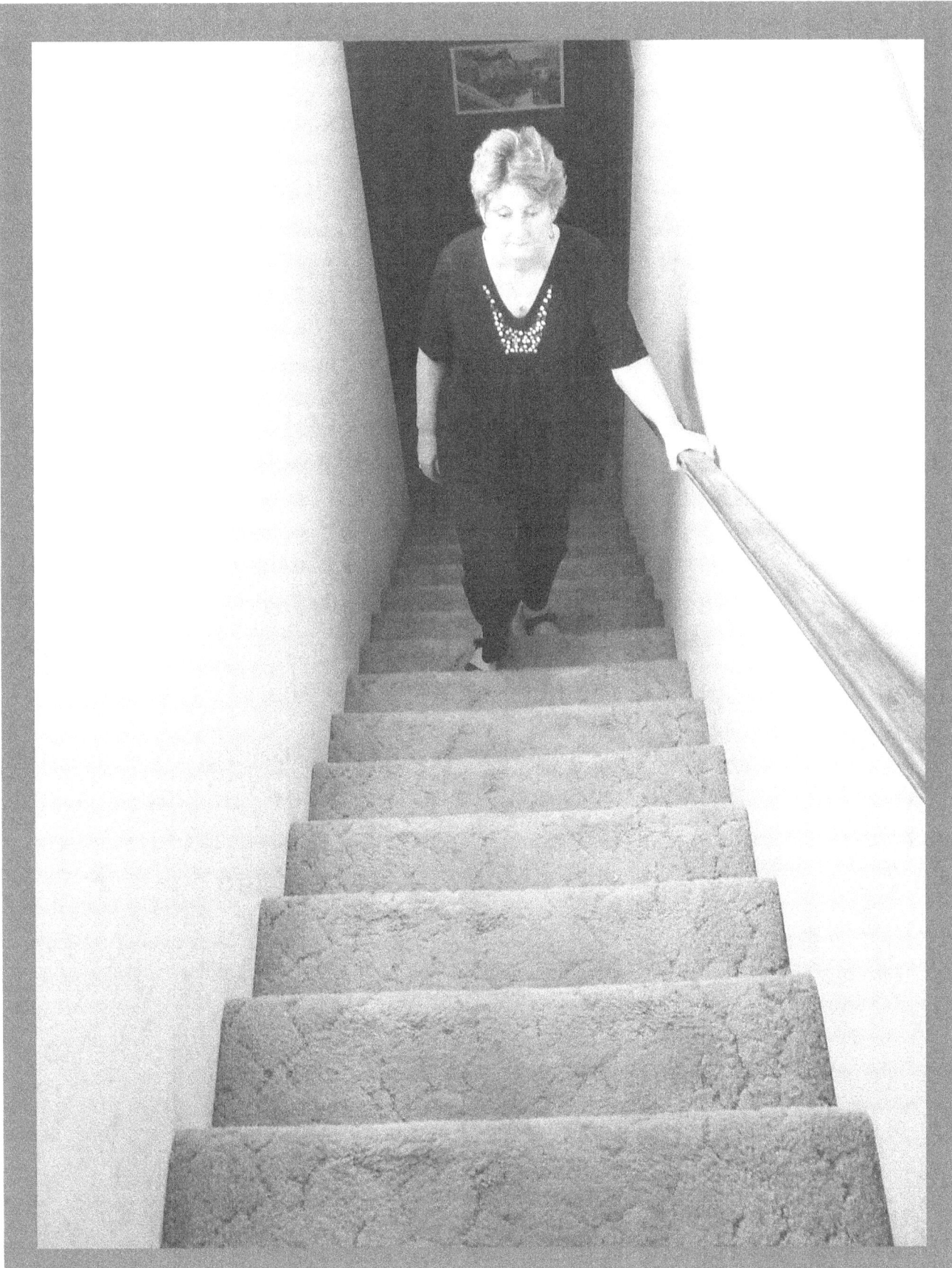

CONGRATULATIONS!

In the time it took to watch a TV show or listen to some music, you've put yourself through stretching and strength-building exercises without having to leave the comfort and safety of your home.

Patience and persistence will lead to great rewards as far as your overall strength and flexibility are concerned. I believe you will see a healthier and happier you; a person who is full of life with a brighter outlook on the future.

There is an old saying. Eat breakfast like a king, lunch like a prince, and dinner like a pauper. Make sure to watch your diet and eat plenty of fruits and vegetables. Monitor your fat, sugar, carbohydrate, and calorie intake and drink plenty of water.

In 2005, I had medical problems partially brought on by my weighing in at 300 pounds. Utilizing many of these same exercises, walking my stairs, and watching my diet, I went down to 225 pounds and excellent blood pressure within one year.

I will admit that there were times when that little voice inside my head told me that what I really needed was a junk-food snack. I actually would argue with it and mention that I wasn't really hungry and that a glass of water or a piece of fruit would do just fine. Eventually that voice bothered me less and less, just as yours will. Do your best to take care of your body and it will do its best for you.

Now, when is that next marathon anyway?

Aloha, and good health to you!

Robert Shaw

ABOUT THE AUTHOR

Robert Shaw started surfing in the 1950s at age nine and, like most surfers, lived a full and exciting life filled with exercise and adventure. As age set in, he surfed a little less and drank more beer, which led to more unhealthy snacks and overeating. Eventually he weighed 300 pounds. After suffering a mild stroke at 56, Robert chose to avoid becoming enslaved to the various medicines that doctors prescribe for high blood pressure, cholesterol, and obesity. After one year of doing these exercises, light weight training, and eating a healthy diet, he dropped 75 pounds and his blood pressure returned to that of a 30-year-old.

Today, at 63 years of age, he still weighs a healthy 225 pounds and is surfing regularly in Hawaii where he has lived with his wife since 1992.

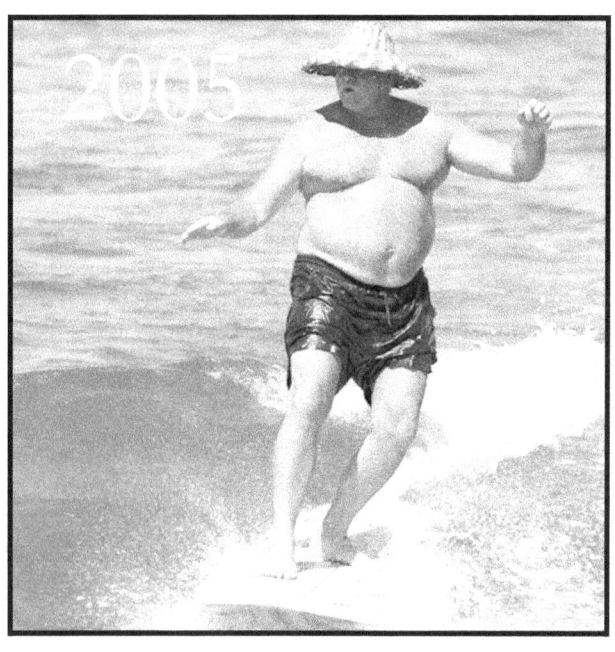 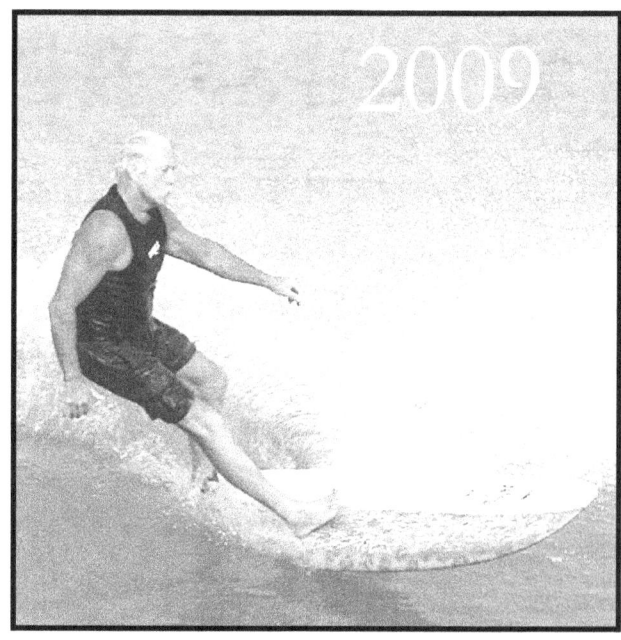

www.ingramcontent.com/pod-product-compliance
Lightning Source LLC
Chambersburg PA
CBHW081401280526
45788CB00009B/2954